A

PRACTICAL TREATISE

ON THE

DOMESTIC MANAGEMENT

AND MOST IMPORTANT

DISEASES OF ADVANCED LIFE.

This is a volume in the
Arno Press collection

AGING AND OLD AGE

Advisory Editor

Robert Kastenbaum

Editorial Board

Joseph T. Freeman
Gerald J. Gruman
Michel Philibert

See last page of this volume
for a complete list of titles.

A

PRACTICAL TREATISE

ON THE

DOMESTIC MANAGEMENT

AND MOST IMPORTANT

DISEASES OF ADVANCED LIFE

GEORGE E. DAY

ARNO PRESS
A New York Times Company
New York • 1979

Editorial Supervision: Joseph Cellini

Reprint Edition 1979 by Arno Press Inc.

Reprinted from a copy in the University of Illinois Library

AGING AND OLD AGE
ISBN for complete set: 0-405-11800-7
See last pages of this volume for titles.

Manufactured in the United States of America

Library of Congress Cataloging in Publication Data

Day, George Edward, 1815-1872.
    A practical treatise on the domestic management and most important diseases of advanced life.

    (Aging and old age)
    Reprint of the 1849 ed. published by Lea and Blanchard, Philadelphia.
    Includes index.
    1. Geriatrics. 2. Aged--Care and hygiene.
3. Home nursing. I. Title. II. Series.
RC952.D39 1979   618.9'2   78-22198
ISBN 0-405-11815-5

A Note About This Book

In his introduction, Day (1815-1872), a Fellow of the Royal College of Physicians, discusses the neglect of the subject of old age in clinical medicine. He had kept notes of his reading, personal observations, and books to produce a practical treatise in which he gave particular thanks to Canstatt. He said "Canstatt's work contains an excellent regimen of everything that had been written on the subject up to the date of its publication" and he utilized that standard work in many ways in his own publication. One major contribution by Day was the collection of a remarkable bibliography, possibly the best that had been put together since the 1804 work of Sinclair. The reprinting of this bibliography is a necessity for students of science. The work divides life into periods of growth, maturity and decline. Most of the first chapter was devoted to the changes that occur during the decline. Rules for the preservation of health, in which the scope of the daily activities were defined, were supported by the chapters in which the common diseases of old age and their treatment were outlined. Each chapter examines diseases of a particular body system with very explicit descriptions.

ON THE
DISEASES
OF ADVANCED LIFE.

A

PRACTICAL TREATISE

ON THE

DOMESTIC MANAGEMENT

AND MOST IMPORTANT

DISEASES OF ADVANCED LIFE

WITH AN APPENDIX,

CONTAINING A SERIES OF CASES
ILLUSTRATIVE OF A NEW AND SUCCESSFUL MODE OF TREATING
LUMBAGO AND OTHER FORMS OF CHRONIC RHEUMATISM,
SCIATICA AND OTHER NEURALGIC AFFECTIONS,
AND CERTAIN FORMS OF PARALYSIS.

BY

GEORGE E. DAY, M.D.,

FELLOW OF THE ROYAL COLLEGE OF PHYSICIANS, AND PHYSICIAN
TO THE WESTERN GENERAL DISPENSARY.

"The reasons why Persons in this age fall so soon into this decrepit state, and why the miseries thereof are so multiplied and magnified upon them, is, because either they call not in soon enough for help, or because those that are called in either understand not, or minde not what they ought to do. An honest and an able Physician may surely approve himself to his ancient Patient *a restorer of life and nourisher of old age.*"

King Solomon's Pourtraicture of Old Age.

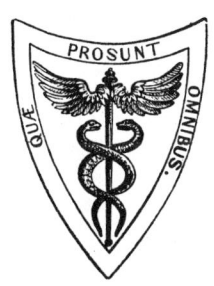

PHILADELPHIA:

LEA AND BLANCHARD.

1849.

TO

JAMES MONCRIEFF ARNOTT, F. R. S.,

VICE PRESIDENT OF THE ROYAL COLLEGE OF SURGEONS,

PRESIDENT OF THE ROYAL MEDICAL AND CHIRURGICAL SOCIETY,

PROFESSOR OF SURGERY AT UNIVERSITY COLLEGE,

AND SENIOR SURGEON TO UNIVERSITY COLLEGE HOSPITAL,

THESE PAGES ARE INSCRIBED,

WITH DEEP FEELINGS OF RESPECT AND GRATITUDE,

BY HIS FRIEND AND FORMER COLLEAGUE,

THE AUTHOR.

INTRODUCTION.

I offer no apology for the publication of this volume. The subject is one of the highest importance, and yet it has been strangely overlooked during the last half century by the Physicians of all countries; for although many valuable essays and monographs on individual points connected with the hygiene and diseases of advanced life lie scattered among the French and German Periodicals, only one systematic work (that of Canstatt) has been written during the period I have indicated.

The want, that I personally experienced, of a standard work on this subject, led me, from the period I entered on the active duties of my profession, to note down for my own guidance, all the facts and observations bearing on the diseases of advanced life and their treatment, which my official connexion with large charitable institutions daily presented to me. I have likewise been in the habit of recording references to all the works, journals, &c., which in the ordinary course of reading I have found to contain any information on these points. The matter that has been thus gradually accumulating from my own experience, and from the records of other labourers in the same field, is now presented to the world in a very condensed form; but, in order to enable others to pursue with greater facility the same subject, or individual departments of it, I have appended to these remarks the bibliography which I have constructed. My great object has been to render this volume an essentially practical work, and with this view I have intentionally omitted any notice of the appearances presented after death from the diseases which I have described in the following pages. This omission will be supplied in a work which will shortly appear.*

* The second volume of Vogel's *Pathological Anatomy of the Human Body.*

With these remarks on the circumstances which have given rise to this volume, I leave it in the hands of my readers. I shall be fully rewarded for the labour I have bestowed upon it, if hereafter I find reason to believe that it has been productive of any practical improvement in the treatment of the diseases of advanced life.

27, *Upper Seymour Street, Portman Square.*
November, 1848.

There are a few points which I accidentally omitted to notice in their proper places, or which have become known to me as the volume was passing through the press.

In my remarks on sleep and sleeplessness in Chapter II., it was my intention to have directed the attention of the profession, and of my readers generally, to the *Patent Spring Bedstead*, or *Rheiocline*, which has been in use in the Medical and Surgical Wards of the Middlesex Hospital for upwards of two years, and is, I believe, also employed in King's College, Guy's, and St. George's Hospitals. For bedridden persons, and for all cases in which a prolonged continuance in bed is necessary, this invention is of great importance. The spring bedstead possesses the following advantages over the waterbed. (1.) It is much more comfortable to the patient; and (2.) it is more salubrious, and does not give rise to the cold perspiration and damp chill of which patients on a water-bed so commonly complain.*

Since I wrote the remarks on sleep and sleeplessness, I have had much more experience in the use of chloroform, and have had opportunities, during a recent visit to Edinburgh, of conversing with Professor Simpson on the subject, and of seeing him administer it in a number of cases. There is no age at which chloroform may not be given with perfect safety, with the view of procuring sleep. In a letter which I have lately received from Dr. Keith, who was formerly Dr. Simpson's assistant, and co-operated with him in the researches which led to the discovery of the anæsthetic properties of chloroform, he informs me that he has successfully given it, with this object, to patients of 76 and 82 years of age. In these cases we need not administer the chloroform to such an extent as to render our patients quite insensible.

I have in some cases administered chloroform in an emulsive draught. It acts first as a carminative, and secondarily as a soporific. The dose is from half a drachm to a drachm; from its pungency it must be prescribed in a considerable bulk of emulsion.

In connexion with the subject of chloroform, I may mention, that it is the best solvent of camphor with which we are acquainted.

---

* These beds may be seen at the inventor's, Mr. Edward Cottam, 76, Oxford-street. Their price varies from five guineas upwards; but for hospitals they are constructed at a lower rate.

One drachm of chloroform dissolves three of camphor. Hence we have a ready means of giving this substance in a fluid form, just as we should give chloroform itself. For this important pharmaceutical discovery, we are indebted to the Messrs. Smith of Edinburgh.*

In the following BIBLIOGRAPHY I have freely availed myself of the assistance afforded me by Canstatt's labours.

* See *The Monthly Journal of Medical Science*, Nov., 1848.

Stromer, *Decreta medica de Senectute.* Norimb. 1537.
Hier. Brisienus, *Geræologia.* Tridenti, 1585.
Anselmus, *Gerocomica, seu de senum regimine.* Venet. 1606. 4to.
Laurentius, *De senio discursus.* Argent. 1625. 12mo.
Sebiz, *Diss. de senectute et senum statu ac conditione.* Argentorati, 1641.
G. H. Welsch, *De senec. et senum statu ac conditione.* Argent. 1655.
J. C. Michaelis, *De senum affectibus.* 1660.
Meibomius, *Tractatus epistolaris de longævis.* 4to. Helmest. 1664.
John Smith, *The Pourtraicture of Old Age.* 2d Ed. Lond. 1666.
Albertus, *Diss. de senectute.* Lips. 1667.
Faseltus, *Diss. de natura senis.* Videb. 1671.
Yon, *Ergo senecta plena malis.* Par. 1673.
De Berger, *Diss. de morbis senum.* Colon. 1673.
Roger Bacon, *The cure of Old Age and preservation of Youth; Tr. Lat.* by Richard Brown, M.D. *Also a physical account of the tree of Life,* by Ed. Mad. Arrais, *Tr. Lat.* 8vo. Lond. 1683.
D. Vesti, *De affectib. senum Salamonis.* Erf. 1692.
Schrader, *Diss. de senectutis præsidiis.* Helmst. 1699. 4to.
Stahl, *Diss. de senum affectibus.* Halæ, 1710.
Glagau, *Diss. de senectute ipso morbo.* L. Bat. 1715.
De Pré. *Diss. de analogia inter prim. et ultim. ætat. in stat. san., morbos et diætet. etc.* Erf. 1720.
Vater, *Diss. de senectutis præsidiis.* Vitemb. 1724. 4to.
R. Welsted, *De ætate vergenti liber, etc.* Lond. 1724.
Floyer, *Medicina gerocomica.* Lond. 1724.
J. Hutter, *Diss. qua Senectus ipsa morbus sistitur.* 4to. Halæ, 1732.
Ranchius, *Gerocomica.*
Bacquere, *Medicus senum.*
Filholt, *De senectute seu de tuenda valetudine in senio.* In Bibliotheca Halleri.
Hoffman, *Diss., qua senectus ipsa morbus sistitur.* Hal. 1732.
Juch, *Diss. de senectute.* Erf. 1732.
Liefman, *Diss. de adynamia artis medicæ in senibus.* Erf. 1737. 4to.
Woeldicke, *Progr.: Cur paucissimi inter homines senescunt.* Hafniæ, 1737.
Ferret, *Quæstio med., an senium a fibrarum regiditate.* Par. 1739. 4to.
Wolff, *Diss. de senectutis natura et artibus longissimam vivendi senectutem veris.* Erf. 1748.
Richard Mead, *On the Disease of Old Age,* in his *Medica Sacra.* Lond. 1749.
Gaille de St. Léger, *Quæst. med., an homini maturo senescere et ultimum mori, tam*

naturale, tam ineluctabile sit, quam adolevisse et maturuisse? *Affirmat.* Par. 1751. 4to.

G. G. Richter, *Progr. de constantia senilis valetudinis.* Gœtting. 1752.

Probstius, *Diss. de hæmorrhag. nar. in senibus.* Hal. 1752.

Gernet, *Diss. de siccitatis senilis effectibus.* Lips. 1753.

G. G. Richter, Resp. J. S. de Berger, *Diss. de sene valetudinis suæ custode.* Götting. 1757. 4to.

De Büchner, *Diss. de plethora senum, etc.* Hal. 1758.

Ludwig, *Progr. de sanitate senili.* Lips. 1759. 4to.

Pollich, *Diss. de nutrimento, incremento, statu et decremento corp. hum.* 4to. Strasb. 1763.

Juncker, *Diss. de causis quibusdam præmaturæ senectutis præcipuis.* Hal. 1765.

J. F. Cartheuser, *De incommodis senectutis.* Francof. 1770.

Behrens, *Epist. gratul. de causis senii.* 1770.

Sam. Farr, *Aphorismi de marasmo ex summis medic. coll.* Altenburg, 1774.

De Fischer, *de senio ejusque gradibus et morbis, etc.* Erf. 1754. *Tr. Lat.* by H. H. Weichardt. Leipz. 1776. Also, in German, under the title of *Abhandl. v. Alter. d. Menschen.* Lipz. 1777. 8vo.

Robert, *De la Vieillesse.* Par. 1777.

J. C. Pohl, Resp. Hænel, *Diss. de morbis ex senio.* Lips. 1777.

Van Swieten, *Oratio de senum valetudine tuenda.* Vienn. 1778. 4to.

Fogerolles, *De senum affectibus præcavendis.*

Benj. Rush, *On the condition of the Body and Mind in Old Age, together with remarks on the Diseases of Old Persons.*

J. A. Unzer, Vol. xii. p. 321.

Triller, *Pr. de senilib. morb. diverso modo a Salamone et Hippocrate descript.* Viteb. 1781.

Premauer, *Diss. de causis præmaturi senii et mortis.* Friburg, 1782. 4to.

Albites, *Disquis. de consequenda et producenda senectute.* 1790. 8vo.

E. Valli, *Entwurf eines Werkes über das hohe Alter.* Translated from the Italian, by S. Bonelli. Wien. 1796. 8vo.

Alibert, *Diss. pour servir de réponse au mémoire du D. Valli.* See *Mémoires de la soc. med. d'émulat. An.* V. T. 1, p. 357.

Stant, *Diss. explicat. aphorism. Hippocratis* 34. sect. 2. Harderov. 1797.

B. G. Seiler, *Anatomiæ corporis humani senilis specimen.* Erlang. 1800.

Const. Anast. Philites, *De decremento altera hominum ætatis periodo, seu de marasmo senili in specie.* Hal. 1808. 8vo.

J. H. F. Antenrieth, Resp. C. L. Essig, *Diss. de ortu quorundam morborum ætatis prodectioris, præcipue opthalmiæ senilis.* Tub. 1806. 4to.

F. H. Simon, *Diss. de infante et sene.* Wirceb. 1806. 8vo.

W. J. Schmitt, *Uber diejen. Krankheiten der Harnblase, Vorsieherdrüsen u. Harnröhre, denen vorzüglich Männer im hohen Alter ausgesetzt sind.* 8vo. Wien. 1806.

R. W. Seiler, *Pr. de morbis senum.* Viteb. 1817. 4to.

Salgues, *Hygiène des Vieillards.* Par. 1817.

A. Carlisle, *Essay on the disorders of Old Age, and on the means of prolonging life.* Lond. 1817. 8vo.

Marshall Hall, *Commentaries on some of the more important Diseases of Females.* Lond. 1824.

BIBLIOGRAPHY.

Jahn, *Ueber die Verwandtschaft der Greises- und Kinderkrankheiten.* (Hecker's *Lit. Annalen.* 4 Jahrg. Oct. pp. 128–155.)

S. T. Sömmering, *Abhandlung über die Schnell und Langsam tödtlichen Krankheiten der Harnblase und Harnröhre bey Männern im hohen Alter.* 2d Ed. Frankf. 1822.

J. B. Foucart, *Quelques observations tendant à prouver l'utilité des emissions sanguines et du traitement anti phlogistique en général dans beaucoup de maladies des Vieillards.* In the *Archiv. Gen.* 1824.

Mayer, *Von den Veränderungen welche die weiblichen Genitalien namentlich der uterus in hohen Alter erleiden.* Bonn. 1825.

G. Breschet, *Note sur l'anatomie des Vieillards,* in the *Archiv. Gen.* 1826.

Halford's *Essays and Orations.* Lond. 1831.

Hourmann et Dechambre, in the *Archiv. Gén.* 1835, &c.

Guyétant, *Le Médecin de l'age de retour et la vieillesse.* Par. 1837.

Canstatt,* *Die Krankheiten des höheren Alters und ihre Heilung.* Erlangen. 1839.

Ant. Friedr. Fischer, *Das Alter und dessen Gebrechen und Krankheiten.* 2d. Ed. 1840. 8vo. Pesth.

Gendrin, *De l'influence des Ages sur les Maladies.* Par. 1840.

Prus, *Mémoire sur les Maladies de la vieillesse* in the *Mem. de l'Acad. Roy. de Med.* 1840.

Holland, *Medical Notes and Reflections.* Chap. xix. *On the Medical Treatment of Old Age.* Ed. 2d. Lond. 1840.

Menville, *De l'age critique chez les femmes, &c.* Paris, 1840.

Raudnitz (L.), *Die Gebrechen des Alters und die Art ihnen zu entgehen, etc.* Prag. 1840.

Dubreil, *Observations sur les aneurismes, etc.* Montpellier, 1842, containing observations on the cause of hypertrophy of the left ventricle in old people.

Röderer, *Ueber die Pneumonie der Alten,* in *Oester. Med. Wochensch.* Jan. 1843.

Newcourt, *Sur l'effet des saisons sur la mortalité des Vieillards,* in the *Journ. de Med.* May, 1843.

Beau, *Etudes cliniques sur les maladies des Vieillards,* in the *Journ. de Med.* Oct. 1843.

Martin, *De la Pneumonie des Vieillards,* in the *Revue Médicale.* Jan. 1844.

Bianchon, *Die Krankheiten der Greise.* Translated from the French. Nordh. 1845.

Vigla, *Sur les symptomes de la pneumonie chez les Vieillards,* in the *Journal des Connaiss. Medico-Chir.* May, 1847.

To these I would add the articles on *Age* by Renaulding in the *Dict. des Sciences Med.*; by Rullier in the *Dict. de Med.*; by Begin in the *Dict. de Med. et Chir. Prat.*; by Roget in the *Cyclopædia of Practical Medicine*; by Copland in his own *Dictionary,* and by Symonds, in the *Cyclopædia of Anatomy and Physiology*: and I would refer the reader to the articles *Senectus* and *Longaevitas* in Ploucquet's *Literatura Medica.*

---

* Canstatt's work contains an excellent *resumé* of every thing that had been written on the subject up to the date of its publication. I have drawn freely from his work in several parts of this volume.

TABLE OF CONTENTS.

INTRODUCTION, Page vii.

CHAPTER I.

Pp. 25–36.

ON SOME OF THE MOST IMPORTANT CHANGES OCCURRING IN THE SYSTEM IN ADVANCED LIFE.

Different periods of human life, 25. Epochs of declining life, 26. Diseases incidental to these epochs, 26. Ill-marked inflammation of a principal organ generally the immediate cause of death, 27. No fear of death in very aged persons, 27. Anatomical changes in the respiratory organs and modification in their functions, 28. Modification in the nervous system and its functions, 31. The insulation of the different organs, 34. Changes in the digestive organs, 34. Causes of dyspepsia, 35. Imperfect formation of blood, 35. Changes in the organs of circulation, 35. Consequences of the heart's action being either too strong or too weak, 36. On the pulse, 36.

CHAPTER II.

Pp. 37–53.

ON THE PRESERVATION OF THE HEALTH IN DECLINING LIFE.

Rules to attain a good old age, 37. Importance of regular habits, 38. Occasional danger of correcting bad habits, 38. Selection of meal times, 38. General rules regarding diet, 38. Application of animal chemistry to cookery, 38. Best method of boiling meat, 39. Liebig's directions for making soup, 40. Broiled and roast meat, 40. Larding, 40. Frying, 40. The best kinds of meat, 40. Milk, 41. The birds used for food, 41. Eggs, 41. The best kind of fish, 41. Turtle, 41. Oysters, 42. The best kind of vegetables, 42. Puddings, 42. Fruit, 42. Ordinary drinks, 42. Beer and ale, 42. Wine, 43. Brandy, 43. Breakfast, 43. Luncheon, 43. Dinner, 43. Tea, 43. Atmospheric influences, 44. Chilliness of old people, 44. Directions regarding dress, 44. Modes of preserving the animal heat in bed, 45. Effect of seasons on the mortality of aged persons, 45. Importance of attention to the skin, 46. Bathing and friction, 46. Anointing, 47. Exercise, 47. Sleep and sleeplessness, 48. (See also page ix. of the Introduction.) Wakefulness, 49. Electricity and magnetism in reference to sleep, 49. Necessity of attention to the excretions, 50. Checked perspiration and how to treat it, 50. Excessive perspiration, 50. The bowels and their proper regulation, 51. Peculiar form of beneficial diarrhœa, 52. Danger of retaining the urine too long in the bladder, 52. Bad consequences of too frequently passing it, 53. Urinary deposits, their utility or danger, 53.

CHAPTER III.

Pp. 53–59.

GENERAL OBSERVATIONS ON THE MEDICAL TREATMENT OF ADVANCED LIFE.

Difference of the effects of age on the two sexes, 54. Two forms of atrophy, the lean and the fat, 54 (note). Absence of reaction in advanced life, 54. How much may be left to nature? 55. Fallacious character of the pulse, 55. Peculiar form of inflammation in old people, 56. Topical bleedings may be combined with tonics and stimulants, 56. Is venesection justifiable in advanced life? 56. Larger doses of medicine often required than in earlier life, 57. The form in which medicines should be administered, 57. Cases in which it is expedient to administer medicines by the rectum, 57. Blisters and other counter-irritants, 57. The medicines of most service in advanced life, 57. Danger of narcotics, 58. Chloroform, 58. Purgatives, 58. Tonics, gum-resins, and balsams, 59. Stimulants, 59. The danger of interference in certain cases, 59. Augmented danger of surgical operations, 59.

CHAPTER IV.

Pp. 60–64.

CLIMACTERIC DISEASE.

The Greek theory of climacterics, 60. Renovation and decay, 60. Progress and symptoms of climacteric disease, 61. Its connexion with other diseases, 62. Reason why it is less common in women than in men, 62. Causes, 63. Treatment, 63.

CHAPTER V.

Pp. 64–66.

SENILE MARASMUS OR WASTING.

The true decay of nature, 64. Symptoms, 65. Treatment, 65. Influence of a nutritious diet, 65. Method of making very strong beef-tea, 65.

CHAPTER VI.

Pp. 66–67.

ON THE DISEASES MOST FATAL TO PERSONS IN ADVANCED LIFE.

My deductions from the Registrar General's Tables, 66. The number of persons dying from sheer old age, 66. Comparative frequency of death from different diseases, 66.

CHAPTER VII.

Pp. 68–102.

DISEASES OF THE RESPIRATORY SYSTEM.

SECTION I.

PNEUMONIA OR INFLAMMATION OF THE LUNGS.

Extreme frequency of pneumonia in advanced life, 68. Probable error in our mortality tables, 69. Causes of pneumonia, 69. Hypostatic pneumonia, 70. Mode of attack, 70. Symptoms, 71. Progress, 74. Prognosis, 74. Treatment, 75. Latent pneumonia, 77. Cases of sudden death from pneumonia, 78.

SECTION II.

BRONCHITIS OR INFLAMMATION OF THE AIR-TUBES.

Early symptoms of bronchitis, 78. Causes, 79. Progress, 79. Prognosis, 80. Treatment, 80. Importance of attention to the humidity of the air in the sick room, 81. Want of tone in the mucous membrane after an attack, 82. Its treatment, 82.

SECTION III.

CHRONIC BRONCHORRHŒA, OR THE MUCOUS FLUX OF THE AGED.

Expectoration common in advanced life, 82. Symptoms, 83. Causes, 83. Progress, 84. Prognosis, 84. Treatment, 84.

SECTION IV.

ASTHMA.

Definition of asthma, 86. Organic asthma, 87. Dry asthma, 87. Humid asthma, 87. Cachectic asthma, 88. Urinous asthma, 88. Symptoms, 89. Gouty asthma, 89. Symptoms, 89. General treatment of asthma, 90.

SECTION V.

HYDROTHORAX AND PULMONARY ŒDEMA.

Hydrothorax seldom a primary affection, 92. Causes of water on the chest, 92. Treatment, 92. Œdema of the lungs, 93.

SECTION VI.

PULMONARY CONSUMPTION AND HÆMOPTYSIS.

A large number of deaths after the age of 60 are ascribed to pulmonary consumption, 93. Case of consumption lasting forty-seven years, 94. Occasional rapidity of the disease in advanced life, 95. Treatment, 95. Hæmoptysis, a less serious symptom than in early life, 95.

SECTION VII.

INFLUENZA.

Nature of Influenza, 96. History, 97. Fatality, 97. The Epidemic of 1847–8, 97. It was most fatal to old persons, and to those suffering from chronic diseases, 98. Its origin, 99. Probably dependent on the presence of ozone in the atmosphere, 99. Method of testing for ozone, 100 (note). Every epidemic presents slight peculiarities, although the more important symptoms are constant, 100. The most obvious symptoms, 100. Treatment, 101.

CHAPTER VIII.
Pp. 103–125.

DISEASES OF THE NERVOUS SYSTEM.

SECTION I.

APOPLEXY AND PARALYSIS.

Fatality of diseases of the nervous system, 103. Different conditions give rise to similar head-symptoms, 103. Hyperæmia of the brain and its symptoms, 103. Danger of confounding Anæmia and Hyperæmia, 104. Symptoms of Anæmia, 104. Head-symptoms from passive congestion, 104. Diminution of nervous energy, 105. All these causes predispose to apoplexy or paralysis, 105. Apoplexy essentially a disease of advanced life, 105. Premonitory symptoms of apoplexy, 105. Necessity for caution in blood-letting, 106. Dangers after an attack, 107. Treatment of the pains occurring in paralysed limbs, 107. Restoration of the suspended nervous function, 107.

SECTION II.

MENINGEAL APOPLEXY.

Remarks on diseases of the serous membranes generally, 108. Premonitory symptoms of meningeal apoplexy, 108. Differences between sub-arachnoid and intra-arachnoid hemorrhages, 109. Diagnosis, 109. Duration, 110. Treatment, 110.

SECTION III.

CEREBRAL SOFTENING.

Cerebral softening is essentially a disease of advanced life, 110. Acute softening, 111. Its symptoms and progress, 111. Chronic softening, 112. Its symptoms and progress, 113. Diagnosis of cerebral softening, 114. Prognosis, 114. Causes, 114. Treatment, 114.

SECTION IV.

MENINGITIS OR INFLAMMATION OF THE MEMBRANES OF THE BRAIN.

A frequent disease of old persons, 115. Points in which it differs from meningitis in earlier life, 115. Symptoms, 115. Causes, 116. Diagnosis, 116. Treatment, 116.

SECTION V.

ON THE MENTAL DISEASES OF ADVANCED LIFE.

The probability of insanity increases with advancing years, 117. Insanity connected with the cessation of the menstrual discharge, with the healing of ulcers, &c., 117. Erotic insanity, 117. Insanity in which moroseness is the predominating symptom, 117. Senile dementia or fatuity, 118. On the gradual decline of the mental faculties, 119. General tendency towards senile dementia, 120.

SECTION VI.

PAINFUL AFFECTION OF THE NERVES.

Neuralgia generally, 121. Comparative frequency at different periods of life, 121. Neuralgia of the fifth pair, Facial Neuralgia, or Tic-Douloureux, 122. Importance of examining the teeth and gums in these cases, 122. Cervico-brachial neuralgia, 122. Dorso-intercostal neuralgia, 123. Sciatica, or femoro-popliteal neuralgia, 123. General treatment of neuralgia, 123.

CHAPTER IX.
Pp. 125–155.
DISEASES OF THE DIGESTIVE TUBE AND ITS APPENDAGES.

SECTION I.

FUNCTIONAL DISEASE OF THE INTESTINAL CANAL—DISEASES OF THE STOMACH.

Relative frequency of this class of diseases, 125. Loss of appetite dependent on weakness, 126. Flatulence, 126. Constipation, 127. Aphthous eruptions of the mouth, 127. Pain and difficulty in deglutition, 128. Water-brash, 129. Senile dyspepsia, 129. The varieties of dyspepsia most common in advanced life, 129. Acute atonic dyspepsia, 129. Follicular gastric dyspepsia, 130. Dyspeptic cough, 131. English cholera, 132. Gastritis of aged persons, 133. Metastatic gastritis, 133. Gouty gastritis, 133. Ulcerative chronic gastritis, 134. Cancer of the stomach, a disease of advanced life, 134. Three stages of the disease, 135. Symptoms of cancer of the stomach, 135. Treatment, 135.

SECTION II.

DISEASES OF THE RECTUM AND ANUS.

Congestion of the rectum, 137. Tendency to abdominal plethora in advanced life, 138. Causes of congestion of the rectum, 138. Symptoms, 138. Hemorrhage from the rectum, 139. Its treatment, 139. Hemorrhoidal tumours, 140. Their treatment, 141. Mucous discharge from the anus, 141. Inflammation of the rectum, 142. Its symptoms and treatment, 142. Itching of the anus, 143. Its treatment, 143. Idea of Dr. Lettsom that it is dangerous to check this itching, 144. Stricture of the rectum, 144. Its symptoms, 144. Treatment, 146. The rectum bougie, 146. Abscess near the rectum, 147. Paralysis of the rectum, 147. Paralysis of the sphincter ani, 147.

SECTION III.

DISEASES OF THE LIVER.

Gall-stones, 148. Symptoms of the difficult passage or impaction of a gall-stone, 148. Treatment, 149. Senile jaundice, 150. Its progress, 151. Treatment, 152. Dropsy of the abdomen, 152. Depends on a stagnant and loaded state of portal circulation, 153. Symptoms, 153. Treatment, 153. Organic dropsy, 154.

CHAPTER X.

Pp. 155–162.

DISEASES OF THE HEART.

The heart often enlarged in advanced life, 155. Functional diseases of the heart, 156. Palpitation, 156. Weakness of the heart's action, 158. Syncope or fainting, 158. Angina pectoris, 159. Neuralgia of the heart, 159. General remarks on organic diseases of the heart, 159. Observations on the anatomical changes generally observed in the heart in old age, 160. Treatment of organic diseases of the heart, 160. Dropsy from disease of the heart, 161. Treatment of dilatation of the heart, 162.

CHAPTER XI.

Pp. 162–187.

DISEASES OF THE URINARY AND GENERATIVE SYSTEMS.

SECTION I.

The various causes of retention of urine, 162. Paralytic retention, 162. Its progress, 163. Treatment, 163. Value of the galvano-magnetic current, and ergot of rye in these cases, 164. Retention of urine from enlargement of the prostate, 164. Symptoms of chronic enlargement of the prostate, 165. Treatment, 166. Enlargement of the prostate from varicosity of its vessels, 167. Retention of urine from inflammation of the bladder, 167. Retention from spasm of the neck of the bladder, 167. Danger of too long a voluntary retention of urine, 168. Chronic inflammation of the bladder, 168. Catarrh of the bladder, 169. Diseases of the kidneys consequent on enlarged prostate, 170. Incontinence of urine, 170. Irritability of the bladder, 170. Bloody urine, 170.

SECTION II.

ON THE DISEASED CONDITION OF THE KIDNEYS ACCOMPANIED BY ALBUMINOUS URINE.

Bright's disease, 171. Sources of Kidney-disease, 171. Symptoms of Bright's disease, 172. Importance of chemistry and the microscope in the diagnosis of urinary affections, 172. Other diseases are associated with this affection, 173. Treatment, 173.

SECTION III.

ON THE DIMINISHED SECRETION OF URINE IN ADVANCED LIFE.

Frequency of this affection, 175. Symptoms, 175. Most marked symptoms are a constant desire to make water, and an irritable state of the skin, 176. Treatment, 177.

SECTION IV.

ON URINARY DEPOSITS, GRAVEL, AND STONE.

The conditions giving rise to the deposition of uric acid from the urine in a concrete form, 178. Symptoms preceding deposits of uric acid, 178. Danger of checking the elimination of uric acid, 178. Causes of these deposits, 179. Diagnosis and prognosis, 179. Other sediments than uric acid or urates, 181. Symptoms and treatment of a concretion on its course from the kidney to the bladder, 181. Age at which stone in the bladder is most common, 182. Reasons why this is the case, 182. Symptoms and treatment of stone, 182–3. Advanced age no bar to lithotomy, 183. Risk of that operation, 184. On the solution or disintegration of stone in the bladder, 184.

SECTION V.

Neuralgia dependent on a morbid condition of the genito-urinary organs, 185. Unnatural excitement of the sexual feelings in advanced life, 186. Premature decay of the reproductive functions, 186. Uterine hemorrhage in advanced life, 186.

CHAPTER XII.

Pp. 187–198.

SECTION I.

DISEASES OF THE SKIN.

The Erythema of advanced life merely a modification of œdematous erysipelas, 187. Chronic eczema, 188. Herpes zoster, 189. Herpes preputialis, 189. Chronic pemphigus, 189. Rupia escharotica, 190. Chronic ecthyma, 190. Impetigo sparsa, 190. Acne rosacea, or carbuncled face, 190. Prurigo, 191. Lichen agrius, 193. Psoriasis, 193.

SECTION II.

ON ULCERS OF THE LEGS.

Danger of too rapidly healing ulcers, 194. Evidence from the writings of Whately, Baynton, and Home, that sometimes the cure of an old ulcer in persons of advanced life is followed by an improved state of the health, 194. Mode of deciding whether interference is advisable, 195. Treatment, 195.

SECTION III.

SENILE GANGRENE.

The parts commonly attacked, 195. Symptoms and progress of the disease, 195. Moist and dry gangrene, 196. Diagnosis, 196. Causes, 196. Treatment, 197.

CHAPTER XIII.

Pp. 198–210.

GOUT AND RHEUMATISM.

Acute gout, 198. Premonitory symptoms, 199. Recurrence of gout, 199. Exciting causes, 200. Treatment of the premonitory symptoms, 201. Treatment during the paroxysm, 201. Value of colchicum, 202. Other remedies, 202. Local applications, 203. Treatment during convalescence, 203. Burdock root, 204. Bitters, Menyanthes trifoliata, Portland powder, 204. Value of sulphur, the Chelsea pensioner, 204. Diet of gouty persons, 205. Chronic gout, 205. Its treatment, 206. Value of local applications, 206. Irregular gout, 206. Illustrations, 206. Rules for treatment, 207. Retrocedent gout, 207. Treatment, 208. Acute rheumatism, 208. Chronic rheumatism, 208. Rheumatic gout, 208. Its treatment, 208. Value of mineral waters, 209.

APPENDIX.

Pp. 213–224.

The importance of the thermic treatment, 213. History of the discovery, 213. Cases illustrative of its value in lumbago, and other rheumatic affections, paralysis, sciatica, &c., 214.

CHAPTER I.

ON SOME OF THE MOST IMPORTANT CHANGES OCCURRING IN THE SYSTEM IN ADVANCED LIFE.

Different Periods of Human Life—Declining Life—Its Epochs—Declining Age—Advanced Age—Mature or Ripe Old Age—Decrepitude or Second Infancy—Alteration in the Structure and Functions of the different Organs—In the Respiratory Organs—In the Nervous System—In the Digestive Organs—In the Organs of Circulation—The Pulse in Old Age—Changes in the Genito-urinary Organs.

HUMAN life is divisible into three great periods—those of Growth, Maturity, and Decline.

During the season of growth all the powers of the system are directed to the building up and perfecting of the different organs constituting the whole body. Although every organ, even to its minutest particle, is undergoing a constant change, yet the supply exceeds the loss, and the body accordingly continues to increase in bulk. In course of time, as the period of growth approaches its close, these antagonistic processes of reparation and decay approximate nearer to an equality, till at length they are exactly balanced.

The system has now reached its state of maturity. There is no longer any augmentation of size or alteration of form. The parts only maintain the *status* they have already acquired. There is however still a continual changing of the particles; the change consisting in the regular formation of new parts to take the place of those which are worn out and removed from the system. For a long series of years, varying in different individuals according to their habits of life, and the original stamina of the constitution, this equilibrium is wonderfully and beautifully retained; but a season ultimately arrives when the beam begins to decline on the opposite side, when the powers of the system can no longer meet the full demands made upon them, when the vital energies begin to give way, in short when the maturity of life almost imperceptibly glides into its decline. The age at which this change commences varies considerably in the different sexes, but it is most commonly observed to begin at about the 40th year in women, and the 48th or 50th in men. It is of the period of life succeeding this change, of the hygienic rules necessary to be observed during it, and of the diseases incident to it, that we have to treat in this volume.

The years of declining life are naturally divisible into the following epochs:

1. Declining age, extending in women to about the fifty-second year, and in men to about the sixtieth.

2. Advanced age, or incipient old age, extending in women from fifty-three to about sixty-five, and in men from sixty to seventy.

3. Mature or ripe old age, dating from the preceding period, and extending to about seventy-five in the female, and eighty in the male.

4. Decrepitude, or second infancy, constituting, in those whose span of existence is so far prolonged, the last epoch of human life.

During the first of these epochs, the feelings, disappointments, and anxieties of life exhibit their effects on the internal organs, as well as on the external appearance, in a more forcible degree than in earlier life. In consequence of the circulation becoming more languid, venous congestions and visceral obstructions, with the various diseases depending on them, become frequent. Piles, apoplexy and paralysis, diseases of the liver, kidneys, and bladder, structural changes in the heart, dropsy, chronic affections of the respiratory organs, gout, and insanity now frequently develop themselves. These affections are common to both sexes; there are however some—and by no means the least important—to which the female sex is alone liable. In this period occurs that great change which indicates the termination of what we may term her active sexual life. Morbid affections of the womb and its appendages, as well of the breast, are now very frequent, being either developed at this period, or having previously remained dormant.

During the second epoch, most of these tendencies increase in frequency and severity. The energies of the nervous, circulating, and muscular systems begin to flag, and languor and feebleness begin to steal over the frame, and impair the activity of the various functions. The faculty of conception ceased in the previous epoch; the power of procreation is now impaired, or even abolished.

During the third period, the above changes are more strongly marked. The teeth fall out, the form of the lower jaw alters, and the digestive functions become much impaired. The peculiar leanness of old age begins now to show itself. Amongst the most common diseases of this period, we may mention a peculiar form of dyspepsia arising from imperfect digestion and assimilation; chronic inflammations, frequently terminating in organic changes, owing to the diminished force of vital resistance; hence probably the frequency of senile gangrene; apoplexy and paralysis, comatose or sleepy affections resulting from declining nervous energy; passive hæmorrhages, indicative of a general want of tone in the system; and disorders of the urinary organs in the male sex.

During the last epoch, all the physical and mental powers rapidly decline. The face is pallid, and devoid of expression; the cheeks sunk, and the eye dim. In consequence of the absorption of the fatty tissue, the skin is lax, wrinkled, and dry. The limbs are feeble; the knees totter and bend under the weight of the body; the trunk stoops and is curved forwards. All the destructive tendencies previously alluded to, continue to act with increasing energy, because the frame is less able to offer any available opposition to them. The "age that melts in unperceived decay" is rarely met with amidst the numerous causes of premature decrepitude, to which civilized man is almost necessarily exposed. I am inclined to agree with Dr. Paris, that in most cases death is immediately owing to an ill-marked species of inflammation in some principal and formerly enfeebled organ.

There is one observation I would yet make before closing these introductory remarks; it is with reference to the views with which aged persons regard their approaching dissolution. It seems as if the earnest desire for life diminished in almost the same proportion as its possession was withdrawn. It is very seldom that old persons regard death with feelings of terror. I cannot call to mind a single instance in which, as far as my own experience extends, a dying person of the age of eighty or upwards has not looked forward to death with pleasure rather than with fear.

I now proceed to the anatomical consideration of the changes most commonly occurring in advanced life. If the fact can be established that at this period the most essential organs present certain fixed peculiarities which modify to a great degree the due performance of their functions, need I adduce a single argument to prove that after these modifications are once established in the system, the progress of ordinary disease must be materially affected, and the processes of treatment modified accordingly?

I shall notice at some length the alterations, in structure and function, of the organs most liable to be affected in old age. These organs are—

  1. The Respiratory Organs,
  2. The Nervous System,
  3. The Digestive Organs, and
  4. The Organs of Circulation.

Modifications in the Respiratory Organs and their Functions.—The osseous case inclosing the lungs and heart is usually altered in form. Its upper portion is flattened at the sides, causing a well-marked diminution of the transverse diameter. The vertical diameter is shortened in consequence of the diminished height of the intervertebral cartilages, and as the anterior portion of these cartilages is most rapidly absorbed, we have forward curvature of the spinal column, as a further cause tending, in conjunction with the others, to lessen the capacity of the chest. The intercostal spaces lessen in size, till contiguous ribs come in contact with one another, and the cases are not rare in which, in extreme age, they are found actually united.

The ribs diminish in density, and lose their elasticity, and the cartilages of the two first are usually ossified. Union of the chondro-sternal articulations is not very common, and the joints uniting the ribs with the spine generally preserve their mobility. The inferior boundary of the thoracic cavity—the diaphragm—is naturally altered in form, in consequence of the preceding changes. We find it thrown in folds, the impressions of which are often well marked on the upper surface of the liver.

The lungs of aged persons vary considerably in their aspect.* These varieties have been comprehended by Hourmann and Dechambre in three typical forms, by which one lung may differ from another, or parts of the same lung from other parts. I have slightly modified their views in a few points.

First Type.—In muscular persons, with a well-formed thorax, not very much altered by the ravages of age, the lungs present little appa-

---

* I have entered fully into this subject, in consequence of its importance in relation to the normal sounds of the chest in advanced life.

rent difference from those of the adult, except in the altered position of the great interlobular fissure. The degree of this alteration corresponds with the extent of lateral flattening. In the adult this fissure lies immediately beneath the upper lobe, and passes obliquely to the root of the lungs, so that on the right side the central lobe occupies exactly the middle part, and on the left side has the lower lobe immediately beneath it. But in old age the fissure approximates to the vertical direction, so that one lobe of the left lung is directly in front, and the other behind, and the middle lobe of the right lung projects downwards, and the lower lobe becomes elevated behind it, so as to form the posterior fourth (or more) of the summit of the organ. On examining a thin dried section under the microscope, the cells are found to be about double the size observed in a similar section of an adult lung.

Second Type.—The lungs are of regular form, but small, light, and hardly capable of being distended sufficiently to fit the thorax even by the strongest inflation, and when thus inflated, the air escapes more readily than from the adult lung. On pressing them between the fingers, the ordinary crepitation is entirely, or for the most part, absent. They are bathed in a clear serous fluid. The cells, on examining a dried section, are found to be larger than in the preceding type, and there is an obvious diminution of the fine vascular tissue that is so apparent in the adult lung.

Third Type.—The lungs lie closely attached to the vertebral column, and form an irregular mass surrounded by much serous fluid. They are livid and flabby, and their normal conical form is no longer recognizable, the summit being often larger than the base. The fissures have sometimes apparently disappeared, and the lobes are merely united by a flat, thin pedicle. Inflation does not much increase their size. They are very light, and communicate to the touch the sensation of a skein of flax. In this case the microscope exhibits cells of a highly irregular form, but of larger dimensions than in the preceding types. Very few vessels are perceptible.

These facts verify the law announced by Magendie, that the density of the lungs diminishes, as also does the quantity of blood they admit, with the progress of age. The thorax gradually accommodates itself to this change ; it becomes atrophied as the lungs atrophy ; it contracts as they contract. The effusion of serum may be owing, at least in part, to the chest being unable to contract beyond a certain point, so that as the lungs diminish, the serum may fill the vacant space.

There is yet another point to be noticed in connexion with the lungs of aged persons, namely, the black deposit which is frequently found in the respiratory organs.* It seems due to the stagnation of the blood in the pulmonary tissues. When it occurs in great abundance it is capable of producing considerable inconvenience by obstructing the capillary vessels and respiratory canals. The absorbents diminish with the advance of old age. The fibrous tissue of the bronchial tubes not unfrequently becomes hypertrophied, and thus lessens their capacity; and their contraction is often much increased by chalky deposits in the sub-mucous tissue, by thickening of the mucous membrane from repeated inflammations, and from various other causes. Ossification of the thyroid and crycoid cartilages, and of the rings of the trachea and bronchi presents an additional obstacle to the free entrance of air.

Let us now consider the modifications in the functions of these organs consequent on the above changes.

As the respiratory organs become worn out, the necessity for employing them seems to diminish in a corresponding degree. The movements of the chest, especially in the transverse direction, are much diminished, and become irregular both in number and in duration. The diaphragm becomes the chief agent in inspiration. The scaleni and sternocleido-mastoidei muscles are rendered almost useless when the spine is much curved; and to remedy this, the head is thrown back at each inspiration, so as to put these muscles to the stretch. Ordinary expiration is sudden and rapid: forced expiration, as in coughing and expectorating, is difficult when there is much curvature, in consequence of the relaxed condition of the recti, obliqui, and transversales muscles. From the examination of 255 women, ranging in age from 60 to 96 years, Messrs. Hourmann and Dechambre† found that the number of respirations in a minute averaged 22.

The diminution in the expansive power of the lungs, and in the extent of exposed mucous membrane, and the decrease of the vascular tissue sufficiently indicate that the changes produced in the blood while passing through the lungs must be very different from those occurring in the adult. The change from venous to arterial blood

---

* See my translation of Vogel's *Pathological Anatomy*, vol. i. pp. 191–193.

† Dr. Pennock found that in 170 men, whose average age was 64·09 years, the mean number of respirations was 20·51, and that in 143 women, of the mean age of 70·57, it was 22·06 in a minute.—See *the American Journal of Medical Science*, vol. xiv. p. 68.

cannot be efficiently brought about. The circulating fluid leaves the lungs with the impress of venosity still adhering to it. The carbon, which ought to be eliminated by the lungs as carbonic acid, is only imperfectly removed, and the corresponding volume of oxygen which ought to be absorbed in its place, and conveyed in the blood to every cell within the organism, carrying with it health and vigour, can no longer gain admittance into the system.

Moreover, the altered state of the vascular tissue and of the bronchial mucous membrane presents an obstacle to the free escape of the aqueous vapour charged with organic matter, which is usually evolved from the pulmonary organs. In consequence of this retention the lungs have a tendency to become œdematous, and the depositions so frequently found in the lungs of the aged are probably in some measure dependent on the same cause. That the character of the pulmonary excreta also varies, is obvious from the fetid odour of the breath, not unfrequently noticed. If the urinary secretion is checked, the breath often has an ammoniacal smell.

Modifications in the nervous system and its functions next claim our attention. We have undoubted evidence that with advancing years the brain diminishes in size, weight, and specific gravity. The same is also the case with the spinal cord, the nerves, and the ganglia of the sympathetic system.

The skull is considerably diminished, owing doubtless in part to the absorption of the diploe. The dura mater adheres to the bone, either universally or at patches, with a degree of tenacity that would be deemed morbid in earlier life: instead of being tensely stretched over the surface of the brain, it presents an appearance of folds corresponding to the deepened cerebral depressions into which it dips. It is frequently penetrated by the pachionian bodies, which often occur in considerable size and large numbers, although they are occasionally altogether absent in advanced life; and sometimes by bony spicula, especially in the portion constituting the falx major. The arachnoid becomes thickened, tough, more opaque, and more of a yellowish white tint than in middle age. The pia mater undergoes corresponding changes; it becomes thicker and firmer, and in consequence of its diminished vascularity assumes a paler tint. We not unfrequently find on it either calcareous deposits, or vesicles filled with fluid or with a mixture consisting apparently of granular matter and cholesterin. The same changes, acting in a less degree, are observable in the membranes of the cord.

There is usually a considerable quantity of fluid in the sub-arachnoid cavity indicating an increase in the space between the surface of the brain and the interior of the skull.

The brain has a shrunken appearance, and its surface exhibits numerous depressions produced by the sinking of the different convolutions. The layer of gray matter covering each convolution is much thinner than in adult life. The convolutions themselves are obviously shrunk, and the sulci between them are much increased in width. The firmness of the brain is usually increased (although cerebral ramollissement is common in old age), so that it admits of being torn in the direction of its fibres, and of yielding a clean section to the knife. The ventricles are dilated and filled with a large quantity of clear, slightly albuminous fluid, varying from two to ten or twelve drachms.

It has been judiciously remarked by a recent writer* on the nervous system, that there is strong evidence tending to show that the occurrence of an increased quantity of fluid, either around the nervous centres or within the ventricles, is a *result*, and that probably *of a conservative kind*, consequent on a change which depresses the general nutrition of those organs.

Its quantity of blood is much diminished; merely a few minute drops of bloody serum start forth from the cut surface, but the open mouths of numerous thickened empty vessels become apparent. The arteries of the base of the brain are almost always more or less diseased. Their former retractile power seems gone, their coats are thickened, opaque, and studded with yellowish white patches, and they usually contain fibrinous coagula; while in adults they contract, and are either perfectly empty or contain fluid blood.

The connexion between the nervous system and the organs of the senses is so intimate, that we shall take this opportunity of noticing the leading modifications which the organs in question undergo.

In the eye the fluids diminish in quantity. The cornea becomes flattened and loses its elasticity. The *arcus senilis* observed around its margin is dependent on the partial obliteration of its nutrient vessels. The iris becomes paler and the pupils smaller. The deep coloration of the choroid coat becomes less intense, and sometimes altogether disappears. The retina becomes more attenuated. The lens flattens, becomes denser, and assumes a pale yellow tint, deep-

---

* Dr. Todd, in *the Cyclopædia of Anatomy and Physiology*. Vol. 3. p. 642.

ening with advancing years. The vitreous humour loses its transparency, and transmits yellowish light. The lachrymal points sometimes close, and there is a continuous flow of tears.

In the ear there is a general hardening of all the structures. The bones of the middle ear unite so as to form only a single piece. The mastoid cells often become filled with bony deposit. The tympanic membrane is tense, hard, and dry; and occasionally is slightly ossified. The cerumen is deficient both in quantity and quality. The fluid of the inner ear is less abundant, and the auditory nerve becomes harder and smaller than in middle life.

The tongue becomes lax and flabby, and its epithelium probably thickens.

The Schneiderian membrane most commonly appears drier than usual; the nose secretes but little mucus, and, as has been already mentioned, the passage for the tears into the nasal cavity is not unfrequently closed.

The epidermis becomes rough, dry, and impermeable, and is obviously no longer adapted to the objects for which it was originally intended. It almost assumes the character of a foreign body, and keeps up a perpetual irritation on the subjacent papillæ in the true skin. We shall notice these changes more at length in the chapter on diseases of the skin.

The functional changes of the nervous system, although less obvious in their origin, are equally well marked. They have been so forcibly described by one of the most classical medical writers of the present day, that I shall transcribe his account of them. "The senses, even without apparent structural disease, lose their power of being excited—become less keen and discriminative. The energy of volition is enfeebled, and its influence over the muscular actions in all ways impaired, often to the extent of partial paralysis, independently of the changes in the muscular tissues themselves. The diminution of irritability and sympathy in all textures of the body, from whatever parts of the nervous system these functions are respectively derived, seems to occur in some ratio to the decline of sensibility and voluntary power. And hence, morbid changes in all the functions of absorption and secretion, on the skin without and the membranes within; and the incapacity of adequately repairing the injuries sustained from accident or disease."*

* Holland's *Medical Notes and Reflections*, 2d edition, p. 286.

In connection with the functions of the nervous system, I would especially direct attention to a point which I believe to be of the highest importance in its bearings on the treatment of the diseases of old age, namely, to what we may term *the insulation of the different organs.* The bond of nervous sympathy, uniting the different organs into one living whole, seems weakened, and in some cases almost snapped asunder. In infancy, from the general sensibility of the system at large, a single lesion will give rise to numerous symptoms. In old age, the symptoms are usually more confined to the morbid organ, and even there they are often masked and obscure. A lung may be perfectly impermeable, or may even be entirely disorganised, yet the heart may afford no indication either by its force or its frequency that one of the most essential of the vital functions is fast ceasing.

If an organ is diseased there is often little or no general reaction, and we do not find, as in earlier life, that one organ can, as it were, come to the rescue of another. Prus has made the following apposite remark on this point: " Enter a ward devoted to the treatment of the diseases of old age, and you will be struck with the thorough indifference with which a patient sees his neighbours die around him: so it is with the economy of old age; the body is destroyed piecemeal without any general reaction, without the appearance of any conservative effort." I need hardly hint at the increased difficulty in forming an accurate diagnosis, that must be induced by this condition of the nervous system.

It hardly falls within the scope of the present volume to follow and trace out the gradual changes occurring in the intellectual functions: such a subject belongs rather to the writer on mental philosophy than on medical practice.

The changes in the *digestive organs* next claim our attention. The first point that strikes us is the diminished capacity of the stomach and intestinal canal, dependent, for the most part, if not altogether on the thickening of the mucous membrane. The muscular coat of the intestines is more or less atrophied, and sometimes not a trace of it is perceptible. The villi and mucous follicles are generally shrunken, and very little mucus is secreted. When we take into consideration the diminished surface of the intestinal tract, the thickened mucous membrane forming as it were a barrier to absorption, the diminution of power in the muscular coat, and the consequent impediment to the peristaltic motion, the imperfect mastication from the partial or entire absence of the teeth, and the modified admixture of the saliva, gastric fluid, bile, &c. (for that these secretions are modified by age, we cannot doubt), we have sufficient reasons to account for the fact of the diminished nutrition of the body in old age. The dyspepsia from which we so frequently observe aged persons to suffer, is probably dependent in part on the prolonged retention of the food in the stomach in consequence of imperfect mastication, in part on the modified state of the gastric juice, but in a greater measure on the blunted sensibility of the nerves of the stomach. There are sound physiological reasons for believing that the flatulence of which old persons so frequently complain is very closely connected with the diminution of nervous power. Let us carry our researches a step or two further. The imperfectly digested food must yield an imperfect chyle; the organs for its elaboration are atrophied, and hence the very source of life—the blood—ceases to be produced in a due and perfect condition, and is, as it were, slowly poisoned at its very birth. One of the sources of the impurity of the blood in old age has been alluded to in our remarks on respiration; another exists in the deficient action of the various glands.

The changes occurring in the *organs of circulation* are at least as well marked as those in the systems we have already considered. The size of the heart and the thickness of its walls, usually diminish with advancing years; occasionally, however, we find that this organ is increased in bulk and power, in consequence of the greater resistance offered by the vessels to the passage of the blood. The lining membrane presents spots of atheromatous deposit, and the free margins of the valves are thickened and much hardened. The arteries contain deposits of calcareous salts and fatty matters,* which deprive them of their proper elasticity, and besides converting them into mere rigid tubes, predispose to rupture of their coats and aneurism. The walls of the capillaries are invariably thickened, rendering the diameter of those vessels smaller; and they seem much diminished in number. I have already alluded to this diminution in the case of the lungs. The pale skin of age contrasted with the ruddy bloom of youth, illustrates the same fact in reference to the skin. The diminished capillaries impede the free passage of the blood from the arteries to the veins; and the propelling force of the heart and arteries being thus deadened, the fluid accumulates in the veins, which consequently become distended and tortuous.

* See the translation of Vogel's *Pathological Anatomy*, Vol. i. p. 584.

In consequence of this derangement of the natural balance of the blood in the different parts of the vascular system, the heart is called upon to do additional work. If it be moderately strong the circulation may be kept up with perhaps no greater apparent deviation from the state of health than piles or varicose veins. If the heart's action be too strong (which is by no means unfrequently the case), the smaller arteries, especially those of the brain, may be ruptured by the force of its impulse, and apoplexy or paralysis may be the result. If the heart be weak, and its action inefficient, there will be a tendency to venous congestions, dropsical effusions, and a general failure of all the functions of the body.

From the ordinary state of the arterial system in old age, we must recollect the uncertainty of the indications afforded by the pulse at the wrist. *The pulse should be counted at the heart.*

Furthermore we must know the average number of pulsations in old age. Physiologists seem to have considered it as an established fact that the frequency of the heart's action diminishes in advanced life. This is a great and dangerous error; I find from the data afforded by 562 healthy women, whose mean age is 73 years, that the average number of pulsations is a fraction above 79 in a minute; and that the average pulse of 197 healthy men of the mean age of 68 years is 72·5. Although the pulse is thus as a general rule above instead of below the pulse in adult life, we not unfrequently meet with cases of very slow pulse in old age. These are, however, exceptional cases.

Such are the most important of the changes illustrating the morbid tendencies of advanced life. There is yet another system—the genito-urinary—in which the changes of structure and function are even more obvious—especially in the female sex. These changes, however, and those occurring in the organs of motion, hardly require a general notice; the former will be sufficiently explained in a future part of this volume, and the latter, in a medical point of view, are of comparatively little importance.

CHAPTER II.

ON THE PRESERVATION OF THE HEALTH IN DECLINING LIFE.

Regular Habits of Life—Meal-times—Choice of Food and Mode of Cooking it—Drinks—Atmospheric Influences—Necessity for Protection from Cold—Fatal Influence of Cold Weather—Necessity for Precaution—Clothing—Attention to the Skin—Bathing—Friction—Anointing—Exercise—Sleep and Sleeplessness—Checked Perspiration—Augmented Perspiration—Attention to the Bowels, and to the State of the Urinary Secretion.

I DEVOTE this chapter to the *hygiene* of declining life—to the consideration of the true means of preserving health. The subject in its general bearings is one of such vast extent, that I must be pardoned if in the opinion of my readers I have passed over some points too briefly.

Man has ever sought to prolong his existence to the utmost extent. Yet how few are there who have not to a greater or less degree shortened the natural term of their life by their own wilfulness and mismanagement. The amount of stamina with which a man is born may do much (and indeed Rush* goes so far as to state that he never met with a person eighty years of age, one or both of whose parents were not long-lived), but the habits of life and the influence of external agents, do far more to determine the years of man's existence.

The rules for the attainment of a good old age are all comprised in a single sentence. *Carefully avoid all such influences as tend to shorten the span of life.* At the present day this may seem so self-evident a truth, as hardly to require or demand the importance I would attach to it. But passing over the extravagant dreams of the adepts, it is scarcely half a century since a distinguished Italian physician proposed to counteract the effects of old age by the administration of oxalic acid, with the view to remove the excess of earthy salts in the system: advocates are still to be found for the transfusion of blood; and an Englishman, professing to be a physician, has, within the last year,

---

* *Medical Inquiries and Observations*, Vol. 2. p. 296.

asserted that frequent small bleedings will ward off old age almost for ever.

Regular habits of life are essential to the well-being of old people. I will even go so far as to assert that in many cases it is dangerous to attempt to correct habits which have an acknowledged pernicious effect. The constitution can no longer adapt itself to a change of circumstances. I have witnessed several cases in which persons at about the age of sixty have become teetotalers, after having drank freely for a period of perhaps thirty or forty years. Few of those men have survived to enjoy the moral benefits of the change for more than two or three years. The same is the case with opium eating.

The above remark holds good with regard to meal-times and the choice of food.

I have no doubt whatever, that the practice of dining early, at from one to two o'clock, is the most conducive to health, in all cases in which persons can afford themselves a couple of hours' rest afterwards. A light supper must then be taken between eight and nine o'clock. In general, however, we find, especially in London, that an early dinner hour presents great inconveniences, and the following hours for meals should then be selected.

> Breakfast between eight and nine.
> Luncheon at one.
> Dinner at five.
> Tea at eight.

I can merely give a few general rules regarding diet. The food of old people should be easy of digestion, and I have found in many cases that they bear made dishes (if not too rich) better than plain boiled or roasted meat. This is undoubtedly dependent upon the greater tenderness of the former.

The following remarks on the chemistry of the kitchen may be useful to many of my readers. So much of the importance of treatment is connected with the due arrangement of the diet, that I feel I am not overstepping the bounds of my professional duty, in endeavouring to explain the rational principles on which the preparation of food should be conducted.

The following observations on the best mode of dressing animal food are deserving of the most attentive consideration. Animal Chemistry has shown that there is a very close analogy between the flesh of all warm-blooded animals.* If flesh employed as food is to form flesh in the body, none of its essential constituents should be extracted by the process of dressing it. To use the words of Liebig, "if its composition be altered in any way, if one of the constituents which belong essentially to its constitution be removed, a corresponding variation must take place in the power of that piece of flesh to re-assume in the living body the original form and quality on which its properties in the living organism depend." In boiling flesh in water, a separation of the soluble and insoluble portions obviously takes place, and this separation is more or less perfect, according to the duration of the boiling, and the amount of water employed. Hence, boiled flesh, when eaten without the soup, contains so much the less nutritious or flesh-making matter, in proportion to the quantity of water in which it has been boiled, and to the length of the boiling.

The following is the best method of boiling meat, and unites all the conditions which give to it the qualities best adapted to its use as food. Place the meat in the kettle or boiler when the water is boiling briskly; a few minutes afterwards add sufficient cold water to reduce the temperature to about $160°$ ($52°$ below the boiling point), and keep the whole at this temperature for some hours. The reason of this proceeding is sufficiently obvious. The juice of the meat contains a large quantity of albumen, a substance chemically identical (or nearly so) with the white of egg. The boiling water into which it is plunged and retained for some minutes, coagulates or stiffens this albumen, at and near the surface, just as if it actually were white of egg. A shell or crust is thus formed which prevents the water from penetrating into the interior of the flesh, and at the same time prevents in a great measure the escape of the soluble constituents into the water; but the temperature is gradually transmitted inwards, and converts the raw flesh into a most nutritious form of diet.

I have shown that the object of immersing meat in boiling water is to prevent the escape of the soluble constituents into the liquid. Now in making soup our object is the very reverse. All the sapid and odorous principles of flesh exist in a soluble state in the meat, and our great aim is to extract them. I shall give the directions of the eminent chemist to whom I have already referred, regarding the manner in which meat should be boiled to yield good soup.

---

* See my note to page 422 of the second volume of the translation of Simon's *Animal Chemistry.*

"If the piece of raw meat be placed in cold water, and then brought *very gradually* to the boiling point, there occurs, from the first moment, an interchange between the juices of the flesh and the external water. The soluble and sapid constituents of the flesh are dissolved in the water, and the water penetrates into the interior of the mass, which it extracts more or less completely. The flesh loses while the soup gains, in sapid matters; and by the separation of albumen, which is commonly removed by skimming, as it rises to the surface of the water when coagulated, the surface of the meat loses its tenderness, becoming tough and hard. The thinner the piece of flesh, the more completely does it acquire the last mentioned qualities; and if in this state it be eaten without the soup it not only loses much of its nutritive properties, but also of its digestibility, inasmuch as the juice of the flesh itself, the constituents of which are now found in the soup, are thus prevented from taking part in the digestive process in the stomach. The soup in fact contains two of the chief constituents of the gastric juice."

Such are the true principles on which soup should be made. The fat must of course be thoroughly removed after it has cooled, and it must then be browned and seasoned.

Broiled and roast meats are generally borne well; and I have no remarks to offer in connection with the processes of broiling and roasting, further than to observe that a mutton chop is rendered more tender and juicy, and therefore more easy of digestion, by cooking it between two others. The central chop in this way escapes any hardening from the direct action of the fire, and retains in the most digestible form all its nutritive constituents.

This process is nearly identical with that of larding, often employed in roasting poultry, &c., by which, as Liebig observes, "the extraction of the sapid constituents from the flesh by its juices, and the evaporation of the water, which causes hardening, are prevented; and the surface, as well as the subjacent parts, are kept in the tender state which is otherwise only found in the inner portions of large masses of flesh."

Frying is an abomination, and should never be resorted to in preparing food for persons who have the slightest regard for the well-being of their digestive organs.

Of the ordinary kinds of meat I regard mutton as the best, and veal and pork as the most objectionable. Salted and very fat meats should be always avoided. Sweetbreads and tripe, if plainly cooked, often rest well upon the stomach. Plain animal jellies are usually admissible.

Milk is a most important article of diet; I have had aged persons under my care whose principal nourishment has been derived for years from this source. At the present time I am attending a gentleman, aged seventy-one years, and who is suffering from dropsy dependent on diseased liver, and from chronic inflammation of the stomach. The only nourishment he can retain on his stomach is milk, with a little lime-water. Whey and butter-milk need never be refused when a patient expresses a wish for them. The cream or butter is the only constituent of milk that is likely to disturb the stomach. The composition, known as Devonshire cream, is very apt to disagree with persons of a dyspeptic or gouty tendency. I have, on one occasion, adopted the suggestion of Dr. Pereira, and prepared an *artificial ass's milk* with advantage. This is done by dissolving a couple of ounces of sugar of milk, in a pint of skimmed cow's milk. I only added, however, half that quantity of sugar.

Amongst the birds in ordinary use as food I would only interdict ducks, geese, teal, and widgeon. Grouse and black-cock sometimes disagree, but I suspect that this most commonly arises from their having been eaten in a state closely allied to putrefaction. For old persons game should be kept till it is tender; but not till it becomes high. I need hardly enter a protest against that insidious poison, the *Pâté de Foie gras.*

Fresh eggs, if not injured by cooking, are nutritious, and easy of digestion. They may be either poached or slightly boiled, so as to coagulate the greater part of the white, without affecting the fluidity of the yolk. A raw egg, beaten up with a glass of sherry and a little sugar, forms with a piece of toast or dry bread, a very excellent luncheon.

The best fish for aged persons and others with impaired digestive powers are whiting, sole, haddock, flounders, plaice, and cod. Turbot is richer and less digestible, but may be occasionally taken—without lobster-sauce. The oily fishes, as eels, herrings, salmon, &c. should be avoided. Dried, salted, smoked, and pickled fish are often highly injurious.

Before concluding the subject of animal food, I would venture to plead for turtle. I believe it to be highly nutritious, and, when plainly cooked, to be easy of digestion, and to be one of the most wholesome kinds of food for persons of weak constitutions. I entertain a similar idea with regard to oysters. I have never seen any bad consequences arise from their use, and patients who have rejected meat and poultry, can frequently take them with advantage. They should be eaten raw, with a little pepper.

Let us turn to the vegetable kingdom. The vegetables most to be recommended are potatoes, turnips, carrots, parsnips, artichokes, vegetable marrow, and asparagus. Peas, beans, and the cabbage-tribe should, as a general rule, be avoided, as liable to induce flatulence. Those who cannot take the above vegetables without melted butter had better abstain from them. Cucumbers must be strictly prohibited; and salads taken with moderation.

Puddings, as a general rule, should be extremely plain. The most wholesome are bread, sago, rice, arrow-root, and tapioca puddings. Rich puddings, and every form of pastry should be carefully avoided.

Fruits must be indulged in carefully. In most cases, when taken perfectly ripe and in moderation they seem serviceable. They should be used at breakfast or luncheon—not after a full dinner. As a general rule fruits are more wholesome when cooked than in their natural condition. I have often found that the bowels of old persons may be better regulated by the use of a roasted apple or a few stewed prunes at bed-time, taken with a little bread, than by any other means. There is one common article of food that would certainly not be used, if its deleterious properties were fully known. I refer to the stalks of the rhubarb plant.* It abounds in crystals of oxalate of lime—the constituent of the most painful kind of stone occurring in the bladder. The same objection holds to the use of sorrel, which is much used in France.

We will now proceed to the consideration of fluid articles of diet—drinks.

I have already spoken of the importance of milk. Its value as a drink is well illustrated by the Swiss, whose principal beverage is milk or whey, and who, as a nation, are remarkable for their longevity. Well-hopped beer, such as is termed *pale ale*, seldom disagrees with hale old people as a dinner-drink. If, however, they

---

* The exact extent to which oxalate of lime in the food tends to the production of mulberry calculus is not yet settled. Most writers maintain the view given in the text; I have, however, shown elsewhere that much depends on the state of the digestive and assimilating functions.—See the eighth of my Lectures *on Chemistry and the Microscope, in relation to Practical Medicine,* in the *Medical Gazette,* vol. 41. pp. 142, 143.

have been accustomed to take water or toast and water at their meals, they had better continue in this practice. As a general rule I have never seen any bad effects from the use of good malt liquors, except in persons of a bilious habit, and in those suffering from a morbid state of the urinary organs.

Vinum lac senum is a very favourite quotation with old gentlemen; and in moderation I fully grant its truth. Those who have become habituated to the use of wine must not have it suddenly withdrawn at a period when any change in the economy of life is hazardous. To those who have not indulged in its use (I do not refer to its abuse), we may well, when the debilities of old age come upon them, say, "Drink no longer water; but use a little wine for thy stomach's sake, and thine often infirmities."

A glass of wine at luncheon, and two glasses at or directly after dinner, may be regarded as about a fair average. The wines I have seen most serviceable are Madeira and Sherry (especially the kind known as Amontillado). Port wine is more likely to disturb the stomach than the others I have named; but I have often found that, from long persistence in its use, and a firm conviction, in the mind of the patient, of its stengthening properties, it would not be wise to advise that it should be relinquished.

A case once fell under my notice, in which the only wine an old lady, aged about seventy years, could take was red Constantia. When it can be obtained in an unadulterated state, it is an excellent wine for old and debilitated persons.

In some few cases I have seen much benefit from the use of a little brandy, mixed with soda-water, as a dinner drink. This proceeding should, however, never be adopted, unless with the concurrence of the physician.

Breakfast should consist of yesterday's bread, or dry toast with a moderate quantity of butter; one or two new laid eggs, lightly boiled, or a little cold chicken or game. Cocoa made from the nibs, or chocolate made with milk and water, may frequently be substituted with advantage for tea or coffee.

Luncheon may consist of a small basin of soup, with a little toasted bread and a glass of Madeira or sherry; or of a sandwich and small glass of pale ale; or of an egg beaten up with a little sherry.

Dinner should be selected from the bill of fare I have already given, and cooked in the manner I have described.

Tea should consist of a couple of cups of tea or coffee, diluted with plenty of milk, and not over sweetened. An excess of sugar is very apt to give rise to acidity.

Those who dine early should take a light supper, corresponding to the luncheon I have described.

To these directions I would add the following:—

Adhere regularly to the same hours. Never eat to repletion. Masticate thoroughly, and eat slowly. Strive against the tendency to fall asleep in your chair after dinner, unless you specially desire to induce an attack of apoplexy.

Persons in advanced life are very susceptible to atmospheric influences. The sources of their own temperature—of their animal heat—are diminished. In youth, and in adult life, the free respiration and circulation, the continuous change in all the tissues and organs of the body, high nervous energy, and abundant muscular motion afford a never-failing supply of heat; but in old age the case is different; the lungs are diminished in volume and in elastic power, the blood-vessels are modified in number and character, and the force of the heart is diminished; the change of tissue is mere waste without a corresponding reparation; the nervous energy is deadened; and muscular motion much lessened. Hence it is that the feet and hands are almost always cold even in healthy old persons, and that they can no longer resist atmospheric influences as they could previously do. It becomes necessary, therefore, that their clothing should be warmer than that of younger persons.* We must prevent the escape of their waning temperature by dresses composed of bad conductors of heat, as flannel and other woolen materials, worn next the skin. These may be worn with advantage three-fourths of the year. If the weather is very oppressive, the flannel may be exchanged for a Jersey or Union-dress, or may be worn over instead of under the shirt or corresponding female garment.

Old persons commonly suffer very much from the cold during the

---

* The servant of the Prince de Beaufremont, who came from Mount Jura to Paris at the age of 121, to pay his respects to the first National Assembly of France, shivered with cold in the middle of the dog days, when he was not near a good fire. The National Assembly directed him to sit with his hat on, in order to defend his head from the cold.

Dr. Rush mentions that Dr. Chovet, of Philadelphia, "who lived to be eighty-five, slept in a baize night-gown, under eight blankets, and a coverlet, in a stove room, many years before he died." It is, doubtless, from the neglect of providing very aged persons with sufficiently warm bedclothes, that they are so often found dead in their beds in the morning, after a cold night.

night. They should be thoroughly warm on going to bed, and in cold weather should sleep with their feet resting upon a stone or tin bottle filled with hot water, and thickly enveloped in flannel. There is, I believe, no measure so influential in supporting the sinking vital energies of age as the communication of animal heat, particularly from the young of our own species. This is one of the oldest* restorative means of treatment practised, having been adopted by King David when he " was old and stricken in years; and they covered him with clothes, but he gat no heat."† Boerhaave caused an old burgomaster at Amsterdam to sleep between two young persons, and we are informed that the old man acquired by this means a visible increase of vigour and activity.

The important influence exercised on the mortality of old people by the temperature of the atmosphere has long been recognised. The remark of Celsus, *senes æstate et autumni prima parte tutissimi*, has been fully verified by statistical observations. The following tables, the first drawn up by Quetelet, and based on 400,000 cases, and the second constructed by myself from the mortality tables of our metropolis, strikingly exhibit this fact.

Ages.	Jan.	Feb.	Mar.	Apr.	May	June	July	Aug.	Sep.	Oct.	Nov.	Dec.
50 to 65	130	122	111	102	93	85	77	85	89	90	100	115
65 to 75	143	132	118	99	91	77	71	80	88	86	98	117
75 to 90	147	139	116	101	87	77	67	75	84	84	100	121
90 and upwards	158	148	125	96	87	75	64	66	76	74	103	129

The total number of registered deaths, at or above the age of 60, occurring in five years (from the first of January, 1843, to the 31st of December, 1847), amounted to 53,048; while the total number of

---

* The following inscription discovered at Rome, in the seventeenth century, seems to allude to this subject.

Æsculapio et Sanita
L. Clodius Hermippus,
Qui vixit annos cxv. dies v.
Puellarum anhelitu.
Quod etiam post mortem ejus
Non parum mirantur physici
Jam posteri, sic vitam ducite.

This inscription gave rise to a very singular work by Dr. Cohausen, entitled, "*Der wiederlebende Hermippus, oder physikal. u. med. Abhand. von der seltsamen Art sein Leben durch das Anhauchen junger Mädchen auf* 115 *Jahre zu verlängern.* 1753.

† 1 Kings, i. 1–4.

registered deaths from age or natural decay, during the same period, amounted to 15,136. Reducing these numbers to a scale of 1000, we have the proportion for each month as follows:—

In 1000 deaths from all causes at 60		In 1000 deaths from old age, unconnected with any obvious disease.	
December	127·0	December	112·3
March	99·8	January	109·6
January	98·8	March	102·3
February	96·1	February	101·0
November	86·7	November	85·3
April	79·3	April	83·2
May	74·3	May	75·3
October	72·5	October	71·4
June	68·2	June	66·4
August	67·9	August	65·2
September	64·8	July	64·3
July	64·6	September	63·2
	1000·0		1000·0

Hence during the colder months those who are far advanced in years should act with the greatest caution, should carefully guard themselves from all atmospheric influences, and should place themselves under the more immediate and constant care of their physician, whose office and duty it is, not only to treat diseases when once established in the system, but to guard his patients from its attacks.

A change of residence to a warmer climate during the cold months, or for a permanency, is often highly serviceable. We are told that when the more opulent of the Romans grew old they were sent to Naples.

A due attention to the condition of the skin is always essential to a state of health. In old age this is pre-eminently the case. The desiccation and death of the epidermis or scurf skin, and the thickening of the cutis can only be prevented by regular ablutions and frictions. The tepid water-bath is an invaluable remedy. The surface of the body must be rubbed by an attendant until a thorough glow is established. In cases where the debility is too great to admit of a regular bath, as for instance when reaction cannot be easily produced, friction must be had recourse to. I regard it as a most important auxiliary to medical treatment, and it is strange that when its therapeutic value is so clearly demonstrated in the writings of the ancient physicians, and is daily exemplified on the sleek skins of our horses, we should have allowed so valuable a practice to fall into almost utter desuetude. Friction may be practised either with the naked hand, with a piece of flannel, or with the flesh-brush. To be of real service the process should be continued for at least half an hour every morning and evening, should be extended not only to the limbs but to the trunk, and especially to the region of the spine, and should be performed by a person properly instructed. In rubbing the abdomen the course of the hand should accord with the direction of the large intestine ; by this simple means we can frequently prevent constipation and relieve the flatulence that is often so distressing in old age.

I was consulted nine or ten years ago by a gentleman between sixty and seventy years of age, for disease of the heart. He had resided most of his life on the continent, and told me that a French physician had advised him to pay especial attention to the condition of his skin. He was provided with an instrument very like the curry-comb we use for horses ; and he stated that if he chanced to omit being curried and rubbed down for a single morning, he always felt the want of his grooming in the course of the day, and was sure to suffer from depression of spirits.

We know comparatively little of the process of anointing. It is probably not of the same value here as in hotter climates, where the oil affords a certain amount of protection against the direct action of the solar heat, and checks the tendency to profuse perspiration. Yet I have no doubt that in many cases it would be found highly serviceable in protecting the skin from the ravages of time and disease. I am glad to find that I have the support of Dr. Holland in bearing me out in this opinion. " There is reason," he observes, " as well as scope, for making larger trial of it as a curative means, even in disorders of the alimentary canal. The harsh dry skin of the dyspeptic patient might be improved in its texture and functions, by rubbing with warm oils, &c., when wholly unaffected by internal remedies, given for the same object."

The classical reader may recollect the answer given to the Emperor Augustus by a hale centenarian, on being asked by what means he had attained to so great an age, and preserved so completely his mental and corporeal powers. " *Intra mulso, foris oleo*," was the reply.

A few words are required on the subject of exercise. Its amount and nature must mainly depend on the strength and previous habits of the individual. Extreme bodily fatigue is highly injurious, and likely to induce the climacteric disease, which forms the subject of a future chapter. Quiet walking, gardening, and riding on horseback, are amongst the most suitable forms of exercise. When only carriage exercise can be taken, the friction applied in the manner described in a preceding page, is advisable, as the best substitute we possess for bodily motion; and of course it is even more valuable when the patient is too infirm to leave the house.

Shortly after breakfast is the best time for exercise, but whenever it is practicable, and the weather is warm and genial, I advise several short periods to be selected. In very fine weather nothing is so effective in warding off after-dinner sleeplessness as a gentle stroll in the open air.

It is difficult to lay down any definite rule regarding the period that should be allotted to sleep. Aged persons should retire early; and should devote from eight to ten hours to repose. If they do not sleep during the whole period (and some old people seem to require little actual sleep), the rest and warmth are highly serviceable to them.

I am very frequently consulted on a point in which medical aid is of comparatively little service—namely, on sleeplessness. Most old people complain of it to a greater or less degree: but I have little doubt that they often deceive themselves on this point. I am told by such persons that they have not closed their eyes for four or five nights—that they slept a few minutes last Wednesday fortnight, and so forth (for extreme particularity in detail is usually observed in these narratives); now in these cases the probability is that they have slept (restlessly, perhaps, and without much refreshment) every night, without being in the least aware of it. I recollect the case of an old woman, a patient at the Finsbury Dispensary, when I was physician to that charity, who used to inform me, in a most piteous tone, that all she required was sleep. I am afraid of saying how long it was since " Nature's sweet restorer" had last visited her, when, calling on her one afternoon, I found her lying on her bed, and sleeping as soundly and comfortably as any old woman could wish to do. The noise of a person entering the room soon after woke her; she rubbed her eyes, looked up, and told me, all she wanted was sleep, that she had not closed her eyes for a month (or some such period), and that if I could not give her something to procure rest, she must infallibly die.

Now, in such cases as these, it is a very bad practice to administer narcotics, and one that should always be avoided if possible. The physician may often do much by insisting on early rising, increased exercise in the open air, and an alteration in the dinner hour, from six or seven o'clock to one or two. A glass of wine, or a little milk with a table-spoonful of old rum in it, shortly before going to bed, may sometimes be prescribed with advantage.

I often find it advisable to recommend a biscuit and a little weak wine and water to be kept at the bedside, and taken during the night. I have found in a great number of cases that old people, who complained that on waking in the middle of the night they could not get to sleep again, have derived remarkable advantage from attention to this point.

During the last few years the disturbing forces of electricity and magnetism have been prominently noticed in reference to the phenomena of sleep. A French physician has written a work with the object of proving that beds should be insulated, which is easily effected by placing the legs of the bedstead on glass blocks; whilst an eminent German philosopher has laid it down as a law that "terrestrial magnetism exerts on certain persons, both healthy and otherwise, who are sensitive, a peculiar influence, powerful enough to disturb their rest, and in the case of diseased persons, disturbing the circulation, the nervous functions, and the equilibrium of the mental powers." Several apparently well-marked cases are described, tending to show that lying in any position except from north to south, is highly disagreeable, but that the position from west to east is almost intolerable to persons sensitive to magnetic influences. The following anecdote, which I quote from Reichenback's Memoirs,* bears on this point. Herr Schuh, a German surgeon, had the singular habit, when he woke early in the morning, which he was invariably in the habit of doing, of turning himself in bed, so as to place his head where his feet had been; on doing this, he invariably fell asleep again, and his second sleep, contrary to the usual opinion, was to him far more refreshing than the whole sleep preceding it. If he omitted this, and lost his second sleep, he felt weary all day, and thus this strange custom had become a necessity with him. His friend Reichenbach found that the head of his bed was directed to the south, and the foot to the north. He advised the turning of the bed into exactly the opposite direction, with the head towards the north, and from that

* See my Report on Reichenbach's Memoir in Ranking's *Half Yearly Abstract of the Medical Sciences*, Vol. 3. pp. 298–302.

time the necessity for the second sleep never returned, the ordinary sleep was refreshing and sound, and the custom above-mentioned at once given up.

This chapter would not be complete were I to omit all mention of the excretions. I have already noticed the importance that must be attached to the preservation of the due action of the skin. We occasionally find cases in which the cutaneous transpiration is so excessive, as to give rise to debility; but, on the other hand, much more is to be feared from the diminution or suppression of this excretion. When the action of the skin is checked by exposure to a cold, damp atmosphere, or to a cutting east wind, by sleeping in damp sheets or remaining in wet clothes, or by any similar cause, the blood is repelled from the surface of the body, and the mucous membranes of the respiratory, and occasionally of the digestive and urinary organs, are very likely (in some old persons quite certain) to become congested, and the congestion too often proceeds to inflammation.

The feelings of the patient will tell him pretty accurately when the skin's action is thus checked, and not an instant should be lost in adopting remedial measures, even before the arrival of the physician. If there would be much delay in obtaining a warm bath, the feet, legs, and hands should be immersed in hot water; and the whole body then vigorously rubbed with hot flannels. This process being concluded, the patient must be placed in a warmed bed ready for his reception, and unless his skin is very irritable, between the blankets. He should then take a cup or two of hot tea or white wine whey, and may afterwards lie snugly tucked up, consoling himself that he has done his best to avert the threatened danger of inflammation of the lungs and bronchial tubes. The sweating usually induced by these steps must however not be allowed to go too far, especially in very infirm persons.

We shall have occasion to return to this subject in the chapter on gout, and in other parts of this volume.

In the cases in which patients complain of excessive perspiration, unless it seems to be debilitating them, I make a point of avoiding all active interference. I have observed this phenomenon most frequently in women a few years after the change of life, and I do not entertain a doubt that it is a salutary effort of nature, perhaps rather to be encouraged than repressed.

Persons who pay little attention to their health in other respects, are apt to expend all their cares and anxieties on their bowels. That the due and regular action of the bowels is of great importance I freely admit, but I much prefer a regular spontaneous action every second or even third day to the continuous use (I should rather say *abuse*) of purgatives. In the description I have given in pages 34 and 35, of the changes occurring in the structures and functions of the digestive organs, the reader will see sufficient reason why the bowels should generally be more torpid in old age than in adult life. It has been my lot to meet with several patients who, from the perusal of popular works on medicine, or from ill-judged professional advice, have felt it an almost sacred duty to obtain, by fair means or foul, a diurnal motion of some sort. I shall notice the bad effects of purgatives in a future chapter, and will therefore only further remark that I have more than once obtained an admission from such patients, after breaking them of this habit, that *they usually felt most comfortable on days when the bowels were not moved.* It is from such confessions as these that the rational physician often acquires his most important knowledge—the knowledge that serves him best at the bedside of his patient; but he, like his patient, is too often the blind follower of an irrational system, and is not easily turned from his idolatry.

If, however, a daily spontaneous action can be obtained, it is far preferable. The importance of punctuality in attention to this office is universally acknowledged, and a moderately early hour is usually recommended. But, forgetting the injunction of an eminent moralist, that "whatever is worth doing, is worth doing well," persons with torpid bowels seldom devote a sufficient space of time to the due completion of the process. If the bowels do not act the moment they are called upon to do so, the attempt is too often at once relinquished, whereas, by repeated gentle contractions of the abdomen, and friction directed along the course of the large intestine (as advised in page 47), the desired object can often be accomplished. Violent straining must be most strictly prohibited. It is liable to induce hernia and apoplexy in persons predisposed to those affections.*

---

* I once, when a student in the Edinburgh Infirmary, saw a man die from this cause. He was suffering from aneurism of the arch of the aorta, which was pointing externally, and it was obvious he could not survive many days. A heavy fall was heard in the water-closet attached to his ward, and on opening the door he was found perfectly dead, lying in his own blood. The effort of straining (and it must have been very slight, for, from the circumstances of his case, every attention was paid to the state of the bowels) severed the last link that united him with the living world.

In my remarks on diet I have noticed certain points bearing on the regulation of the bowels. The intelligent physician will be at no loss to suggest many others. A large draught of cold spring water taken on first rising will often aid the action of the bowels, and can never be productive of harm.

Further observations on this subject will be found in Chapter IX., under the head of *Constipation*.

I have met with several cases in which old people have sought advice for too relaxed a condition of the bowels. The state to which I refer is altogether distinct from diarrhœa. The bowels are moved three, four, and even five times a-day, the evacuations being usually of a pasty consistence, and not assuming a definite shape. If there is no pain on pressing the abdomen, and the tongue has a natural appearance, no active treatment is advisable; a little dietetic management is all that is requisite.

There is only one other point to which I would direct attention in reference to the intestinal excretions, and that is to the common occurrence of watery evacuations from the bowels, resembling those of active diarrhœa, and taking place without any apparent cause, three or four times in the year. They are attended with no distress, and are obviously an effort of nature to purify the system.

I have been frequently consulted by a lady, now in her eighty-seventh year, for an affection of this nature, which she has had for the last twenty-five or thirty years. With the exception of more or less debility, she feels lighter and more cheerful after an attack. If it continue more than two or three days it is expedient to adopt mild medical treatment to restrain it.

The urinary functions, although less under the control of the patient than those of the bowels, claim a passing remark. Aged persons should carefully avoid retaining their water too long. Distended beyond a certain point the bladder refuses to act, and if surgical aid is not speedily procured, death is the sure consequence. So died the illustrious Tycho Brahe. Riding in the same carriage with the Emperor of Austria, he esteemed court etiquette above the mandates of nature, and like all who oppose her insuperable laws fell a victim to his temerity.*

---

* Although not bearing on the special subject of the work, I may mention, as a warning, a most distressing case that occurred a few years ago in a family I have occasionally attended. A young lady setting out with her husband on her wedding tour, was induced from feelings of delicacy to abstain from evacuating

If on the other hand middle-aged or old persons get into the habit of not retaining the urine for a sufficient length of time, the bladder diminishes in size, its walls thicken, and after a time it will not bear the slightest degree of distension, imposing upon its possessor (as a French writer on old age observes) "la necessité de la vider à chaque instant, et déranger tous les actes de la vie sociale."

The urine of old persons generally exhibits a deposit after standing some hours. The nature of these deposits is fully explained in my other works.* I would only observe that in some cases much harm is done by attempting to check the formation of these sediments, this discharge often serving to eliminate from the system matters which, retained in it, would become the source of active disease.

The utility or danger of these urinary deposits is a point on which it is impossible for the patient to judge for himself.

CHAPTER III.

GENERAL OBSERVATIONS ON THE MEDICAL TREATMENT OF ADVANCED LIFE.

Difference of Sex in Relation to Disease—Absence of Reaction in the Diseases of Advanced Life—Danger of trusting too much to Nature—Fallacy of the Pulse in Relation to Diagnosis—Importance of a thorough Knowledge of the Constitution—Peculiar Form of Inflammation in Advanced Life—Treatment of Local Congestions—Blood-letting and its Limitations—Observations on the Mode of Administration of Medicines, and on the Choice of Remedies—Danger of Interference in certain Cases—On the Performance of Surgical Operations.

I PROPOSE in this chapter to notice certain general principles which are of essential importance in the treatment of the diseases of advanced life, and which, I have had occasion to observe, are too seldom duly estimated in ordinary practice.

the bladder till she retired for the night. From its over distension, the bladder was no longer subservient to the summons of the will—in short, was paralysed. Not possessed of sufficient moral courage to communicate her state to her husband, rupture of the distended organ ensued, and in twenty-four hours she was a corpse.

* See my translation of Simon's *Animal Chemistry*, vol. 2, pp. 173, &c.; and my Lectures *on Chemistry and the Microscope, in relation to Practical Medicine*, in the *Medical Gazette*, 1847-8.

Do we sufficiently consider the difference in the effects of age on the two sexes? Women, after they have got through the critical period following the cessation of menstruation, their system having again attained, as it were, a state of equilibrium, generally find themselves better than in the earlier periods of their adult and middle age. Their nervous system loses the irritability which it exhibited as long as the generative functions continued active, and with advancing years becomes more fixed and uniform in its action.

In the male sex the opposite holds good. There is no definite period at which generative excitement ceases, and the changes occurring in advanced life, as, for instance, enlarged prostate, and often more or less stricture, and irritability of the bladder, tend to keep up a degree of morbid excitement, that is in itself almost a disease, and is most prejudicial to the well-being of the individual. I am inclined to believe that it is in consequence of this difference in the condition of the sexes in old age, that we so much more frequently see fat old women than fat old men.*

Another point is the absence of reaction in old age. This is doubtless connected with the deadened sensibility of the nervous system at this period of life. I have given cases in Chapter VII., in which persons in apparent health have died suddenly, and their lungs have been found after death to be in a state of intense suppuration; and yet this morbid process, which must have been going on for some time, had

---

* I extract the following remarks from Mr. Paget's invaluable Lectures on Nutrition, Hypertrophy and Atrophy.

"Atrophy is a uniform concomitant of the infirmities of old age, but the results of senile atrophy are not the same in all; rather you find among old people—you might almost divide them into two classes—the lean and the fat; and these, as you may see them in any asylum for the aged, personify the two kinds of atrophy I have spoken of.

"Some people, as they grow old, seem only to wither and dry up—sharp featured, spinous old folks, yet withal wiry and tough, clinging to life, and letting death have them, as it were, by small instalments slowly paid. Such are the "lean and slippered pantaloons," and their "shrunk shanks" declare the pervading atrophy.

"Others—women more often than men—as old and as ill-nourished as these, yet make a far different appearance. With these, the first sign of old age is, that they grow fat; and this abides with them till, it may be, in a last illness, sharper than old age, they are robbed even of their fat. These, too, when old age sets in, become pursy, short-winded, pot-bellied, pale, and flabby; their skin hangs, not in wrinkles, but in rolls; and their voice, instead of rising "towards childish treble," becomes "gruff and husky."—*Medical Gazette*, vol. 40, p. 144.

not, in any obvious degree, disturbed the ordinary functions of life. Softening of the brain may proceed to a great degree without any obvious symptom. And in the post-mortem examinations of old persons generally, it is no uncommon thing to find grave lesions which were totally unlooked for, in consequence of their having given rise to no functional disturbance. (See page 34.)

This condition of the system increases to a great degree our difficulties in diagnosis and treatment.

In the diseases of advanced life it is often difficult to decide how much must be left to the *vis medicatrix naturæ*. Whilst it is undoubtedly wrong to interfere actively in cases where irremedial changes, depending on the modifications which the system undergoes in old age, have occurred, we must, at the same time, remember that nature can no longer strive successfully with disease as in early life, and that delay in treatment is consequently more dangerous.

At this period of life we derive comparatively little information from the pulse, regarding the intensity and character of the disease, partly in consequence of the absence of reaction, to which I have already referred, and partly to the changes that frequently occur in the arterial system. (See pp. 35, 36.)

These changes often give to the pulse a degree of hardness, which might lead an inexperienced practitioner to suspect acute inflammation. We may, however, ascertain to a certain degree to which cause the hardness is to be attributed, by observing the effect of strong pressure on the character and number of the pulsations. We should, moreover, as I have already remarked, draw no conclusions from feeling the pulse in the ordinary manner. We should contrast the pulses in the radial arteries with those in the temporals and carotids, and especially with the strokes of the heart (see p. 36), which unless much modified by organic changes, affords the most sure criterion of the degree of vascular action. It is, on many accounts, a point of the highest importance to be thoroughly acquainted with the constitution of our patients—to know and examine them in health as well as in disease; for it is on relative rather than absolute differences that we have to found our judgment. Thus, in a person whose average pulse was as low as 50 (and I have had several patients in whom this has been the case), an acceleration to 70 in a minute would indicate as great a degree of vascular excitement, as a pulse of 100 or upwards would do in a person with a pulse naturally rather quick. Cases are recorded by distinguished observers (Morgagni and Rush, for instance), in which regular intermittence occurred in health, and disappeared during disease. These illustrations are sufficient to show the great advantages of knowing the character and number of the pulsations, previous to the occurrence of disease.

These considerations on the pulse lead us to the subject of inflammation and antiphlogistic treatment, especially blood-letting. The physical conditions of the system in advanced life are strongly opposed to the progress of regular inflammatory action; there is, however, a condition dependent on venous congestion, that gives rise to symptoms that in many respects closely simulate it, and that are being daily mistaken for it. These symptoms, however, arise from want of tone and power in the circulating system, and are connected with local plethora, arising from a deficiency of power to propel the blood forwards. Hence, while endeavouring to remove the local stasis, we must carefully avoid any generally depressing treatment. Slight topical bleedings, either by leeches or cupping, may be advantageously combined with remedies of a tonic and slightly stimulating character, given with the view of equalising and improving the tone of the circulation. Venesection is not to be thought of. In these cases the lancet is more fatal than the disease.

Is the use of the lancet ever justifiable in the diseases of old age? It would be highly unphilosophical to assert dogmatically that venesection should never be prescribed after a certain age—whether that age be sixty, seventy, or eighty years—when we know the extreme differences in vigour and constitutional power that old persons of the same age are in the habit of presenting. It is a measure that must be adopted with extreme caution and comparative limitation. We must not only recollect that abstraction of blood is a loss, that in advanced age cannot be easily replaced, but we must bear in mind that numerous cases are on record, in which immediate injury, and even death, have resulted from the practice. When symptoms present themselves, which seem to indicate the necessity for venesection, we must be influenced, in respect to the extent to which it can be borne, by observing the effect that is produced *directly on the heart's action*, not merely on the radial pulse.

The observations I have made on the association of stimulants and tonics with local blood-letting are equally applicable here; in fact, I believe there are very few cases in which Fischer's* advice, that a

---

* De Senio ejusque Gradibus et Morbis, 1754. p. 128.

small glass of good wine should be administered before the operation, may not be advantageously followed. I have only further to remark, that the universal rule that venesection, when absolutely required, should be promptly had recourse to, is especially needful in old age.

There are several points in the therapeutics of old age which I consider of sufficient importance to claim a notice in this chapter.

In consequence of the torpor of the whole system and the debility of the assimilating organs, we often find that larger doses are required in old age than in middle life. This however is not a universal rule.

It is by no means a matter of indifference in what form medicine is administered to old persons. Medicines in a fluid form are preferable to pills and powders, the latter of which are especially apt to disturb the stomach, whilst the former often wend their way through the tortuosities of the intestinal canal, and leave the system in just the same state as they entered it.* The effects of the torpidity of the system are best counteracted by combining the active ingredients with aromatic waters or oils, with bitter tinctures, or with wine.

It is sometimes more advisable to administer medicine by the rectum than by the mouth. This is especially the case in diseases of organs situated in the immediate vicinity of the rectum, as in those of the urinary and generative system.

The peculiar condition of the skin (see page 33), renders the endermic method of treatment comparatively inert in advanced life. Blisters and other counter-irritants are of extreme value in the diseases of old age, but their application requires care, because in consequence of the diminished vitality of the external parts—those most distant from the central organ of circulation—they may give rise to very intractable sores, and even to gangrene.

With respect to the medicines of most service in old age, it may be remarked that the acids and alkalies, although we often find it advisable to prescribe them, should not be given in large doses, or continued for any length of time. The neutral salts must be prescribed with caution. They diminish the plasticity of the nutrient fluid, and if taken constantly are apt to weaken the digestive organs.

---

* I have frequently seen compound colocynth pills pass through the system in this way, and the same is often the case with Plummer's pills if they have been kept for any length of time. In the writings of the early physicians we read of an *everlasting pill*, which was supposed to exert the property of purging as often as it was swallowed. A single pill would thus serve a whole family during their lives, and might be handed down to their posterity as an heir-loom.

On whatever part of the system we wish to act, whether on the intestinal canal, kidneys, skin, or lungs, it is better, when possible, to obtain the desired effect by other means. Nitrate of potash is considered by some physicians to be especially injurious to old people.

The metals are not of very general application at this period of life, and must be prescribed with caution. It is much more difficult to get the system under the influence of mercury than in middle life, and it sometimes produces anomalous and very dangerous effects. The salts of lead are equally objectionable. Iron, antimony, and zinc are often imperatively required, but their administration must be conducted with much more care and moderation than in earlier life. I have never seen any inconvenience from the administration of bismuth.

Iodine and iodide of potassium are not well borne; they give rise to febrile disturbance, and sometimes even to senile marasmus. The same remark holds good for bromine and bromide of potassium.

Sulphur is a highly valuable remedy in old age. It relieves venous congestion, improves the condition of the blood, and exerts a salutary influence on the skin and the pulmonary and intestinal mucous membranes.

It is often a difficult point in practice to determine to what extent narcotics are admissible. From our knowledge of the state of the system in narcotic poisoning, we are aware that the changes which these medicines induce are such as must be injurious in advanced life, and may give rise to cerebral congestion, apoplexy, &c. It is a happy circumstance that at this period narcotics are less required than in earlier life. Instead of the irritable and excitable state of the nervous system, which calls for their employment, we more commonly observe a paralytic tendency, requiring a perfectly different treatment.

There are however numerous cases in which narcotics are requisite, although it is impossible to lay down any general rule on the subject. In the eneuresis of old age, and in some of the most distressing forms of skin-disease, much relief is frequently obtained from them. I have often found the resinous extract of the Cannabis Indica agree with patients who could not bear any preparation of opium.

Chloroform when freely diluted with atmospheric air may often be administered with advantage in painful affections of the nervous system.

As a general rule, presenting however numerous exceptions, we should avoid the use of drastic purgatives; when it is requisite to prescribe them they should be combined with a tonic or stimulant.

In cases where large doses of calomel, Jalap, colocynth, and gamboge have had little more effect than to irritate the intestines, a small dose of the compound gentian mixture, or a few drachms of infusion of senna, with decoction or a little tincture of bark will often be found to act freely on the bowels.

The vegetable tonics, bitters and astringents, and the gum-resins and balsams are amongst the most important articles of the materia medica in advanced life.

Stimulants, as for instance the preparations of ether and the etherial oils, the ammonia salts, phosphorus, and camphor, are now of more value in the treatment of disease, than during the earlier periods of life. I place very great reliance on the therapeutic value of camphor ; and, as far as my experience of so recent a preparation goes, prefer it in the form of Murray's Fluid Solution, of which one ounce contains three grains.

I will conclude this chapter with a few remarks on the propriety of *non-interference* in certain cases.

We are very frequently consulted respecting discharges which are annoying and perhaps alarming to our patients, but which are undoubtedly established by nature as safeguards to the constitution. I may quote as illustrations the profuse discharges from the mucous membrane in senile catarrh and other chronic bronchial affections, certain deposits in the urine, the discharges from the bowels to which I have already alluded, and various passive hemorrhages incidental to advancing years, as epistaxis, hæmaturia, and hemorrhages from the bowels or uterus.

The same remark applies to the rapid cure of long-standing abscesses and skin-diseases, and the removal of issues, setons, &c.

The changes in the system to which I have alluded in Chapter I., and the deficiency in reparative power, render surgical operations more dangerous than in earlier life. We must dissuade aged persons from the very operations, that at a former period we should have advised them to submit to ; and attempt a palliative treatment rather than expose them to the increased risk resulting at their time of life from the shock of the knife. For instance, in cases of hydrocele, the temporary freedom from discomfort which we can yield by a simple puncture is to be preferred to the chance of a radical cure by an operation, which may give rise to great disturbance in the system.

When, as a matter of necessity, great operations must be performed, it is of especial importance to pay due attention to the temperature of the room.

CHAPTER IV.

CLIMACTERIC DISEASE.

The Greek Theory of Climacterics—Renovation and Decay—Progress and Symptoms of Climacteric Disease—Causes—Treatment.

It was supposed by the ancients—and there seems good reason for the supposition—that in passing through life there are particular epochs, at which the body is peculiarly affected, and suffers a marked alteration. These epochs were regarded by the Greeks as five in number, and were named climacterics, from the word κλιμαξ. They begin with the seventh year, which forms the first climacteric; and are afterwards regulated by a multiplication of the figures three, seven, and nine, into each other, as the twenty-first, the forty-ninth, the sixty-third, and the eighty-first years. The two last were called grand climacterics, and it is of the change taking place at or between these epochs, that we have to speak in this chapter. It is of two distinct and opposite kinds—that of renovation, and that of decay. That a sudden renovation of power occasionally occurs in advanced life is an undoubted fact. Cases are recorded by numerous writers, of aged persons who have been deaf for twenty years, suddenly recovering their hearing, so as, in some cases, to hear very acutely; of others as suddenly recovering their sight, and throwing away their spectacles, which had been in constant use for as long a period, and, again, of others in whom there has been a regeneration of teeth and hair.*

---

* The following case recorded in Dr. Rush's Tract on Old Age, rests on the authority of his brother, Jacob Rush, of Reading, in Pennsylvania.

"An old man of eighty-four years of age, of the name of Adam Reffle, near this town, gradually lost his sight in the sixty-eighth year of his age, and continued entirely blind for the space of twelve years. About four years ago his sight returned, without making use of any means for the purpose, and without any visible change in the appearance of the eyes, and he now (June 23, 1792) sees as well as ever he did. I should observe that, during both the gradual loss and recovery of his sight, he was in no ways affected by sickness, but, on the contrary, enjoyed his usual health."

CLIMACTERIC DISEASE.

But, on the other hand, we much more frequently see a sudden and inexplicable decline of the vital powers. And it is to this decay that the term *Climacteric Disease* has been given by the late Sir Henry Halford. That accomplished physician describes it as a falling away of the flesh in the decline of life, without any obvious source of exhaustion, accompanied with a quicker pulse than natural, and an extraordinary alteration in the expression of the countenance.

" Sometimes," he observes, " the disorder comes on so gradually and insensibly, that the patient is hardly aware of its commencement. He perceives that he is sooner tired than usual, and that he is thinner than he was; but yet he has nothing material to complain of. In process of time his appetite becomes seriously impaired; his nights are sleepless; or if he gets sleep, he is not refreshed by it. His face becomes visibly extenuated, or perhaps acquires a bloated look. His tongue is white, and he suspects that he has a fever.

" If he ask advice, his pulse is found quicker than it should be, and he acknowledges that he has felt pains occasionally in his head and chest, and that his legs are disposed to swell; yet there is no deficiency in the quantity of his urine, nor any other sensible feature in the action of the abdominal viscera, excepting that the bowels are more sluggish than they used to be.

" Sometimes the headache is accompanied with vertigo; and sometimes severe rheumatic pains, as the patient believes them to be, are felt in various parts of the body, and in the limbs; but on inquiry these have not the ordinary seat, nor the common accompaniments of rheumatism, and seem rather to take the course of nerves than of muscular fibres.

" In the latter stages of this disease, the stomach seems to lose all its powers; the frame becomes more and more emaciated; the cellular membrane in the lower limbs is laden with fluid; there is an insurmountable restlessness by day, and a total want of sleep at night; the mind grows torpid and indifferent to what formerly interested it; and the patient sinks at last, seeming rather to cease to live than to die of a mortal distemper."

Such is the ordinary course of this disorder in its simplest form when it proves fatal, and the powers of the constitution are unable to counteract its influence. It is seldom, however, that we can observe it in an uncomplicated state, and never, perhaps, but in a patient whose previous life has been entirely healthy, and whose spirits have not been depressed by prolonged cares and anxieties.

It is generally engrafted on other complaints, assuming their character and accompanying them in their course. It blends itself with the effects of any fixed organic mischief in the constitution; takes on the appearances of any periodical irritation to which a patient may have been subject, or adopts the features of a casual disease. When it is associated with organic mischief, it is difficult to distinguish the climacteric complaint from that train of symptoms which commonly supervenes, sooner or later, on diseased structure; but its presence ought to be suspected if the complaints are all unusually exasperated, if a fatal result be threatened earlier than is usual in the common course of things, and above all other indications, if that character be impressed on the countenance which peculiarly distinguishes this disorder.

There is hardly a disease at this period of life with which it may not connect itself. If, for instance, it be engrafted on a common cold, the catarrhal symptoms will continue, and even predominate throughout the greater period of the duration of the climacteric disease, and thus conceal from the patient and his friends the real danger, until, at length, the extraordinary protraction of the complaint, and an unusual decay of flesh and strength, obtrude the painful truth that there is some deficiency of vital power in his system.*

It has been observed that this disease is less common to women than to men. This may be owing to two reasons: (1) that men lead

---

* The following cases appear to be good illustrations of this disease, engrafted on a previous affection. They are recorded by Pinel, and occurred at the Salpêtrière.

A woman, aged 84, was in the infirmary for more than eight months, in consequence of chronic bronchial catarrh with very abundant expectoration and a straining cough. She kept up pretty well during the autumn and the first half of the winter. Towards the end of January the cough became weaker and a state of progressive feebleness ensued. She died about the end of February "sans agonie, sans effort, comme une lumière qui s'eteint."

A woman, aged 81, suffered for a long period from a profuse mucous discharge from the vagina, and from chronic bronchial catarrh. If by any chance the vaginal discharge was diminished, the bronchial symptoms—the cough and expectoration—were always aggravated. In the month of December, without any apparent cause, there was a perfect suppression both of the expectoration and of the vaginal discharge; the features were much altered, the nose pinched, there was deadly pallor, no muscular motion or attempts to move in bed, no appetite, and the urine and fæces were passed unconsciously. She remained in this state for about three weeks and died without a struggle.

a more exhausting and tumultuous life than women ; and (2) that the change which the female constitution undergoes at and immediately after the cessation of the catamenia may render subsequent alterations less perceptible.

Amongst the immediate causes to which this malady may owe its commencement, there is none, according to Sir Henry Halford, more frequent than a common cold. When the body is predisposed to this change, any occasion of feverish excitement, and a privation of rest at the same time will readily induce it. He states that he has known cases in which an act of intemperance, where intemperance was not habitual, was the first apparent cause of it; and I have witnessed cases in which a fall that did not appear of consequence at the moment, and which would not have been so at any other time, has jarred the frame into this disordered action. It may be caused by a marriage contracted late in life ; it may occur on the retrogression of a cutaneous eruption ; but by far its most common cause is anxiety of mind and sorrow. The loss of a wife or husband assimilated to each other in habits and disposition, by an intercourse of perhaps more than half a life, is a more marked and more frequent cause than any other. It is a shock often too great to be borne, and under which the system cannot rally.*

Those who have had most experience in this disease must fain confess that medicine will generally be found to be of comparatively little service. The debility must be met by tonics, cordials, and a generous diet. All exciting causes should be most carefully excluded, and the patient should be led as much as possible to spend his time in agreeable occupations and amusements. For the torpor of the stomach and digestive organs the warmer purgatives, as rhubarb, guaiacum, and aloes, may be prescribed. Quinine, with a stimulating gum resin, may be advantageously united with aloes, in the form of

* The following case—one out of a number that I might quote—will serve to illustrate the point :—A gentleman, aged about sixty, lost his wife, who was a few years younger, from the effects of pulmonary consumption. They had lived happily together for two-thirds of their lives, and he had nursed her with the greatest care and assiduity during the whole of her lingering illness. He was fully aware of her hopeless condition, and in a few weeks after her death seemed almost to have recovered his ordinary spirits. About a month after this, his spirits became again depressed, and he began to lose flesh. His nights were restless, and there was a little fever. The emaciation continued to extend, and in less than six months from his wife's death, he fell a sacrifice to his affections. There are few of my readers but must have seen these distressing cases.

pill. The compound decoction of aloes, and the compound gentian mixture are also useful medicines in these cases. Whatever would weaken the general system must be carefully avoided, and any occasional congestions must be attacked by local rather than general evacuations.

When there seems a tendency on the part of the system towards recovery, the Bath water is often found of much service, particularly if the stomach has been weakened by intemperance, and still more especially if symptoms of gout shall have been blended with those of the climacteric disease.

I would again repeat, that all the so-called lowering treatment in this affection can lead only to one end—the infallible destruction of the patient.

Having already drawn so fully on Sir Henry Halford's valuable essay on this disease, I cannot refrain from concluding in his own words:—

"For the rest 'the patient must minister to himself.' To be able to contemplate with complacency either issue of a disorder which the great Author of our being may, in his kindness, have intended as a warning to us to prepare for a better existence, is of prodigious advantage to recovery, as well as to comfort; and the retrospect of a well-spent life is a cordial of infinitely more efficacy than all the resources of the medical art."

CHAPTER V.

SENILE MARASMUS OR WASTING.

By the term atrophy or marasmus, I mean to imply a wasting away—whether of a single organ or of the whole system—from a mere deficiency of nutrition, and independently of ulceration, morbid deposition, &c.

In this chapter I use it in its general sense, as applying to the whole body. Senile marasmus, as a special disease, finds its place in most of the larger systems of medicine, and in the tables of "causes of death." It is, however, not so much a disease as the gradual wasting of the system—the true decay of nature.

Under the influence of senile marasmus, the desire for food is almost lost; after partaking of it there is a feeling of more or less weight and pain in the region of the stomach; and vomiting is not unfrequent afterwards. There is seldom any unpleasant taste in the mouth; and the tongue either remains unchanged, or is of a bright-red colour, and dry. No hardness or swelling is perceptible in the abdominal region, nor is it tender on pressure.

The evacuations from the bowels are dry, hard, and scanty; and there is frequently great constipation. The least exertion is followed by extreme depression; the emaciation increases; and the pulse becomes very small and weak. At last the patient is confined to his bed, from a feeling of intense debility. Then we usually observe, if not earlier, more or less febrile irritability towards evening. The palms of the hands and the soles of the feet burn, and the cheeks are flushed; the powers of life are gradually and almost imperceptibly extinguished, and at last, without a struggle, " the dust returns to the earth as it was; and the spirit returns unto God who gave it."

We can alleviate the symptoms. We cannot cure the disease, for it is the natural disease of death.

The impaired state of all the organs engaged in the process of nutrition renders it necessary to give the most nourishing kinds of food. Strong soups, animal jellies, plain turtle, oysters, &c. are amongst the most suitable articles of diet. The following is the best mode of making a very strong and nourishing beef-soup—the ordinary beef-tea of the sick-room.

Take 1lb. of lean beef, free from fat, and separated from the bones, in the finely chopped state in which it is used for beef-sausages or mince-meat; mix it gradually with its own weight of cold water, and slowly heat it, till it boils. When the liquid has boiled briskly for one or two minutes, strain it through a thick cloth or towel. In this way we obtain about a pint of most aromatic soup, of such strength as cannot be obtained, even by boiling for hours, from a piece of flesh. It should be of the colour of dark sherry, and may be drank warm or cold.

The extract of flesh obtained by the careful evaporation of the above soup is one of the most excellent restoratives we possess. Its use is, however, apparently unknown to the great mass of practitioners.

Good old wine is highly serviceable, and may either be taken alone, or in a little arrow-root or sago. Sometimes half a glass of Madeira shortly before dinner seems to increase the appetite; the appetite is, however, so capricious in many of these cases, that we must almost break through all regular meal-times, and let our patients eat whenever they express any desire to do so.

The strictly medical treatment must usually be confined to the administration of mild vegetable tonics, and to the due regulation of the bowels.

CHAPTER VI.

On the Diseases most fatal to Persons in Advanced Life.

In the first chapter I mentioned incidentally many of the affections to which the changed state of the system rendered persons of advanced life especially liable. We must bear in mind that there is a wide difference between the most common and the most fatal diseases. It is of the latter that we are now treating. On referring to the Registrar General's tables for the last five years—from 1843 to 1847 inclusive—I have found (see page 45) that the total number of deaths of persons aged 60 or upwards, occurring in the Metropolis during that period, amount to 53,048. Of these 15,136, or about two-sevenths, are recorded as dying from the effects of old age. I have no doubt that if a proper examination after death was always insisted on, this number would be wonderfully lessened, for very few die from sheer old age. But taking these numbers as we here find them, there are left 47,912 cases of death from actual disease.

Death is ascribed to disease of the respiratory organs in 12,598 cases; to diseases of the nervous system in 6947 cases; to diseases of the digestive system in 3141 cases; and to diseases of the circulating system in 2841 cases.

Besides these we have 1076 recorded cases of diarrhœa, 748* of influenza, and 417 of erysipelas.

The following table gives the comparative frequency of the causes of death at and after 60.

Of 1000 persons who have attained that age, there die of old age . 285·3

Diseases of the respiratory organs
- Bronchitis . . . 79·3
- Asthma . . . . 62·4
- Consumption . . . 35·7
- Pneumonia . . . 27·1
- Hydrothorax . . . 10·4
- Other diseases . . 22·6

237·5

---

* Of these, 508 occurred in the last five weeks of the year 1847. During the whole of the four preceding years the total number amounted to 175.

Diseases of the nervous system	⎧ Apoplexy	53·0	⎫
	⎨ Paralysis	51·2	⎬ 130·9
	⎩ Other diseases	26·7	⎭
Diseases of the digestive system			59·2
Diseases of the circulating system	⎧ Diseases of heart	51·3	⎫
	⎨ Pericarditis	1·3	⎬ 53·5
	⎩ Aneurism	0·9	⎭
Diarrhœa			20·3
Influenza			14·2
Erysipelas			7·8
			808·7
Other diseases			191·3
			1000·0

The remaining 191·3 in the 1000 is made up in a great measure of cases of typhus and dropsy (neither of which have been tabulated by me, because the former is made to include all cases of continued fever, and because the latter is a symptom and not a disease, and may arise from very different sources); of cases of diseases of the urinary organs, of cholera, dysentery, cancer, gout, rheumatism, &c.

I shall to a considerable extent adopt the arrangement exhibited in the above table, that is to say I shall commence with the consideration of the diseases of the respiratory organs, and then treat in succession of those of the nervous, digestive, and circulating systems; the diseases of the genito-urinary organs and of the skin will then claim our attention, and the volume will conclude with the diseases of uncertain or variable seat, as gout, rheumatism, &c.

I wish it to be distinctly understood that it has not been my object to write comprehensive essays on the various diseases to which I have just referred. All that I have attempted to do has been to explain the modifications that advanced life impresses on the different symptoms, and to point out the peculiarities in the mode of treatment that should be adopted during the declining period of the vital power.

CHAPTER VII.

DISEASES OF THE RESPIRATORY SYSTEM.

SECTION I.

Pneumonia or Inflammation of the Lungs—Its Causes—Mode of Attack—Symptoms—Pain in the Side—Difficulty of Respiration—Cough—Expectoration—Signs afforded by Percussion and Auscultation—Characters of the Pulse, Skin, and Tongue—Pain in the Forehead—Progress of the Disease—Prognosis—Treatment.

ALTHOUGH pneumonia would not seem, from the position it occupies in the table given in pp. 66, 67, to deserve the first place among the diseases of the respiratory system, there are in my opinion sufficient reasons for giving it the precedence I have here assigned to it. In the first place I do not entertain a doubt that a careful examination after death would have revealed the presence of this disease in a large number of those whose death has been ascribed to bronchitis. My attention was first directed to the extreme frequency of pneumonia in advanced life, by a memoir published about ten years ago by Prus. In the examination of the bodies of 390 persons at the Bicêtre, whose ages ranged from 60 to 90 years, death was found to be dependent on diseases of the respiratory organs in 149 cases.

There were 77 cases of pneumonia, 6 terminating in abscess of the lung.
,,   26   ,,   pleurisy.
,,   18   ,,   tubercular consumption.
,,   10   ,,   asthma.
,,   8   ,,   bronchitis.
,,   4   ,,   pulmonary congestion.
,,   3   ,,   asphyxia from meteorism dependent on indigestion.

The remaining four were isolated cases of comparatively rare disease.

Now, if in the actual examination of 390 bodies, made uninterruptedly for the space of three years (from October 1st, 1832, to October 1st, 1835), it was found that the deaths from pneumonia were to those from bronchitis, nearly as 10 to 1, we are justified in presuming, that in all probability there is an enormous error in our Mortality Tables (which are not based on post-mortem examinations), where, instead of standing at 10 to 1, they stand in the singularly opposite ratio of nearly 1 to 3. For the better illustration of the difference between the Paris and London results, we may place them thus:—

In Paris the deaths from pneumonia are to those from bronchitis in the ratio of 10 to 1; while in London they are in the ratio of 10 to 30.

My own observations, and those of several professional friends, whose attention I have directed to this subject, are strongly confirmatory of the views of Prus. It is, I fear, too often the case, that in old persons this disease is first detected in the dead-house, and if not sought for there, is altogether unrecognised, and the fatal result ascribed to bronchitis, or some equally or more incorrect cause.

Such is the principal reason of my placing pneumonia at the head of the diseases of the respiratory system. Another reason is, that it affords the best illustration of the modifications in treatment, which the inflammatory diseases of advanced life require at the hands of the physician; and on this account, no less than for its intrinsic importance, I have entered into the consideration of this affection more fully than I should otherwise have done.

The *causes* of pneumonia may be divided into the predisposing and the occasional or exciting. The most active predisposing causes seem to be habitual bronchorrhœa, and the constant congestion so regularly observed in the lungs of the aged. A catarrh will often merge into a latent pneumonia, which will run a rapid and unsuspected course, the only evidence of the disease being perhaps afforded after death. Amongst the less direct causes are the rigidity of the frame-work of the organs of respiration, organic diseases of the heart and large vessels, distention of the abdomen, especially from gas accumulated in the intestines and pressing up the diaphragm, and, lastly, debility from age. In reference to age as a predisposing cause, Prus observes, that in the Bicêtre, the cases of pneumonia (from 1832 to 1835) formed nearly one-ninth of all that occurred, and gave rise to nearly one-sixth of the deaths; while Grisolle found, on collecting the facts afforded by the Parisian hospitals for three successive years, that in adult life the cases of pneumonia were to those of the other diseases of that period of life, in the ratio of about 1 to 16, and that the deaths from this disease did not form above one-tenth of the whole mortality. The most important of the occasional or exciting causes are certain conditions of the weather. Although pneumonia may occur at every season of the year, it is especially a disease of the cold months. From a table of 296 cases, collected by Grisolle, without reference to age, it appears that 265, or very nearly nine-tenths, occurred in the seven months extending from the beginning of November to the end of May, while of 156 cases of pneumonia in old women, recorded by Hourmann and Dechambre, 140, or as nearly as possible the same proportion, occurred in the above-mentioned period; of 88 deaths in these 156 cases, 77 occurred during the seven cold months. Sudden changes of temperature, and dry and strong winds, especially those from the north and north-east, seem favourable to the development of pneumonia.

There is another occasional cause, which, with a little care, may often be avoided. I refer to the lying for a length of time in one position. This gives rise to congestion of the most dependent part of the lungs, and is thus a cause of a species of pneumonia, which was first noticed by Piorry, and to which he gave the name of hypostatic pneumonia. This, however, is not a true inflammatory affection.

Mode of attack.—I have not yet been able to satisfy myself regarding the relative frequency of any precursory symptoms in the pneumonia of the aged. Grisolle believes that after the seventieth year such symptoms never present themselves. Hourmann and Dechambre, on the other hand, observe, that in the Salpétrière, the pneumonia occurring in the spring was preceded for several days, and sometimes even for a week or two, by headache, deafness, catarrh with epistaxis, flying muscular pains, &c. My own observations lead me to the belief, that although the patient commonly experiences a feeling of discomfort for a day or two before the disease becomes apparent—in fact, during the period of incubation—there are generally no very distinct precursory symptoms.

There are two distinct forms in which pneumonia makes its attack. If we exclude from our consideration persons with any affection of the heart or brain, it appears that in rather more than half, the attack is acute and scarcely differs from a corresponding attack in earlier life, whilst in the remainder it is obscure and latent.

In the first form it often begins with a shivering fit, which must be regarded as an important symptom. In an adult person, a shivering fit occurring in a state of apparently good health, may be a forerunner of various affections to which old age is not liable, as of numerous forms of fever, acute rheumatism, &c.; in an aged person such a phenomenon should always afford a hint to the physician to look out, and be prepared for pneumonia. Another early symptom frequently preceding and associated with the former, is pain in the side. Although neither the shivering, nor the pain in the side, so frequently precede pneumonia in advanced as in adult life, their presence, when they do occur, must be deemed the more important.

What are the *symptoms* when pneumonia is once established? We can adopt no better mode of classifying them than that adopted by Grisolle, and shall notice (1.), the symptoms presented by the respiratory apparatus, and (2.) the general and sympathetic symptoms.

1. *Symptoms presented by the Respiratory Organs.*—Pain in the side is well known as a symptom of this disease. Its intensity and frequency seem much the same as in adult life, although Hourmann and Dechambre state, that in most of the cases occurring in the Salpêtrière, the seat of pain was indefinite, being sometimes in the whole of the chest, sometimes over the whole of the affected side, but especially anteriorly. This pain is sometimes increased by the slightest pressure. With respect to dyspnœa, our patients often complain of no difficulty of respiration, and sometimes the movements of the chest seem in no degree modified. In other cases, these movements are very irregular, both in force and frequency, and the face presents an appearance of anxiety. Pneumonia of the apex gives rise to more dyspnœa than pneumonia of the base.

Cough is a symptom not much to be relied on; although generally present, it is sometimes so slight as not even to attract the attention of the patient himself. The expectoration differs in some degree from that occurring in the pneumonia of adults. In four patients, whose ages exceeded seventy, Grisolle observed that the sputa were more or less coloured and viscid, but that the colour was less marked than in earlier life. In seventeen out of the sixty-seven cases observed by Hourmann and Dechambre, the sputa were bloody; when they did not contain blood, they presented a gray opaque appearance; and in some few cases they were transparent and viscid. Expectoration[*] is sometimes entirely absent, and often, when it occurs, its

---

[*] There is a peculiarity in ordinary pneumonic sputa noticed a few years ago by Remak in the *Charitie* at Berlin, and which, I believe, I was the first to describe and figure in this country (see *The British and Foreign Medical Review*, vol. 23,

presence is of very short duration. Bloody expectoration is most common in those cases which begin very acutely.

Percussion affords some of the most valuable signs in relation to the diagnosis of pneumonia; it must, however, be borne in mind, that in percussing the chests of healthy old people the sounds differ considerably from those emitted by the chests of adults. Thus when the lungs are in the third type of Hourmann and Dechambre's classification (see p. 29), the sound on percussion resembles that in well-marked emphysema. Again, the region corresponding with the inner half of the clavicle is dull, in consequence of the black depositions usually present in the upper part of the lungs, and of the increased curvature of the clavicle; and the diminished size of the lungs frequently causes a comparative dulness in the sternal region. Bearing these points in view, and recollecting that the differences in the sounds elicited by percussion are merely *relative*, we can interpret these physical symptoms. In the first stage the sounds on percussion are more modified than in the adult, but from the remark I have just made regarding the natural percussion-sounds at this period of life, we must consider a sound as dull in the aged, which would be regarded as clear in the adult. Hence, for the same reason, hepatization does not produce the absolute dulness we meet with in the adult. The dulness is always most marked posteriorly. In the first stage of pneumonia it often happens that, when the ear can detect no difference of sound on percussing similar points up both sides of the chest, the sensations of relative elasticity and resistance conveyed to the finger will indicate the diseased lung.

The remarks I have made, regarding the modified percussion-sounds, apply also to those furnished by auscultation. Independently of disease, we find that when the lungs are in the second type, respiration gives rather a blowing sound than a murmur—a sound compared by Hourmann and Dechambre to that produced by expelling the air through the compressed lips; and when the lungs are in the third type, this sound is so increased as almost to resemble general

---

pp. 504–507), which seems hardly to have met with the attention which it deserves. I refer to the presence of the ramifying bronchial coagula. The earlier the expectoration of the coagula commences, and the more abundant and continuous it is, the more certain and speedy will be the cure. Although these coagula were detected by Remak in every case of pneumonia (his observations embracing fifty cases), yet in four cases of genuine bronchitis, he could not discover the slightest trace of them.

bronchial respiration. Its intensity is very variable, the respiratory sound at one moment being noisy, and perhaps at the next hardly audible. The resonance of the voice is loud, and approaches in character to bronchophony. Let us now inquire how these (which we may term the natural) auscultatory sounds are modified in pneumonia.

The crepitation so characteristic of the first stage of pneumonia in adults is here very rare; it is usually replaced by a sub-crepitant rhonchus depending on the passage of air in larger bubbles and through more fluid, and originating in the increased size of the pulmonary cells, and the general tendency to mucous discharges from the pulmonary mucous membrane of the aged. This sound is usually mixed with, and always succeeded by, bronchial respiration, which is often accompanied by considerable gurgling. The resonance of the voice is not so constantly associated with the bronchial respiration as in the adult, and it not unfrequently approximates in its character to œgophony. Feebleness of the respiration, or its complete absence over a certain extent, combined with bronchophony, are sometimes the only stethoscopic signs; and they may be regarded as affording a pretty certain indication of the disease.

In relation to the auscultation-sounds, I have only to add, that there is undoubted evidence to show that in old people pneumonia occasionally passes through all its stages without giving rise to any perceptible morbid sounds.

2. *General and sympathetic symptoms.*—In old persons affected with pneumonia the pulse is a less trustworthy guide than in earlier life; not unfrequently it is small, intermittent, or irregular. In some cases, where the inflammation is most acute, no change is observable in the frequency of the pulse. The observations relating to the average number of pulsations in advanced life must not be forgotten. There is sometimes a hardness about the pulse in these cases, leading the unwary physician to prescribe venesection, or even its repetition. The hardness and resistance, to which I refer, cannot be reduced by such means; they are altogether, or for the most part, dependent on the peculiar condition of the aged heart. The skin is, at first, usually hot and dry, and either remains in that state till death, or becomes cold, still continuing dry. Sometimes the patient is bathed in perspiration; and in some few cases the skin retains its normal temperature throughout the whole disease. The general febrile reaction is less marked than at an earlier period of life. The tongue varies in its characters.

It is at first white and dry, but as the disease progresses often assumes more or less of a blackish appearance. The digestive organs are generally more or less disordered, and if a dry tongue presents a yellow or brownish coating, we may regard it as an indication of considerable hepatic derangement. In pneumonia of the apex, the face *almost invariably* presents a jaundiced tint. There may be either constipation or diarrhœa; the latter becomes sometimes permanently established after the use of purgatives.

In old persons, as in adult life, pain in the head, most commonly the forehead, is almost constantly present, and this is most commonly followed by more or less disturbance of the intellectual faculties; sometimes there is slight delirium, which usually increases towards the evening; sometimes a condition of stupidity, from which it is almost impossible even for a minute to rouse the patient, supervenes; and this is occasionally followed by coma. The face presents a flushed and livid appearance, which is usually most distinct on the side corresponding to the inflamed lung; as the disease progresses, the redness is replaced by a dusky, and almost earthy tint.

The *progress* of pneumonia in old people is very rapid. In this point of view there is however a singular difference between the duration of the cases terminating fatally and that of those recovering. The mean duration of thirty-three cases that recovered was fourteen days; while in seventy-six fatal cases the mean duration was only seven days (Hourmann and Dechambre.) Sometimes however the disease runs on slowly and unperceived. In very old persons we can seldom achieve a perfect cure. A slight cough and a certain amount of bronchial respiration are persistent, or often supervene on apparent recovery.

The termination of pneumonia in abscess seems more common than in middle life; pleuritis may terminate in empyema.

The *prognosis* is highly unfavourable; Grisolle states that after the seventieth year pneumonia is most commonly fatal, and that although he has seen recoveries in persons exceeding eighty, such cases are extremely rare. Of 129 cases treated by Prus (the ages varying from 60 to 90 years) seventy-seven or about three-fifths terminated fatally. Chomel's practice, as reported by Leroux, affords singularly strong evidence that the peril increases with the patient's age.

The cases between the ages of

13 and 30 were 182, of which 17 or about 9 per cent. died.
30 and 40 ,, 58 ,, 15 ,, 26 ,,
40 and 50 ,, 47 ,, 16 ,, 34 ,,
50 and 60 ,, 55 ,, 23 ,, 42 ,,
60 and 70 ,, 16 ,, 9 ,, 56 ,,
70 and 80 ,, 6 ,, 5 ,, 83 ,,

Hourmann and Dechambre, from their experience at the Salpetriere, describe the frequency of the deaths in pneumonia as 'vraiment effrayante.' Having thus shown that the ratio of mortality to the number of cases seems to vary directly with the age, I shall briefly notice a few of the symptoms on which we should found our prognosis in individual cases. Extreme difficulty of breathing and abdominal respiration are always bad signs. Lividity of the countenance, the struggle for breath, the incapacity to expectorate, a small pulse, disturbance of the intellectual faculties, loud rattles over the chest, and a cold sweat, taken collectively, afford pretty certain evidence of the near approach of death. The free expectoration of thick yellow sputa is regarded as a favourable symptom.

It now only remains to speak of the most appropriate *treatment* of this fearful disease. Is venesection advantageous or even justifiable in the pneumonia of the aged? The stronger evidence lies in its favour, but it must not be had recourse to without fear and trembling. Morgagni took blood from a nonagenarian; P. Frank bled a man aged 80, with pneumonia, no less than eight times during his illness, and the patient recovered; Grisolle states that in ten persons whose age exceeded 70, there was only one who could not stand venesection. Copland states that he has prescribed venesection in two persons between 70 and 80 (in one of them twice), in whom delirium, a symptom usually regarded as contra-indicating blood-letting, was present, and that they both recovered quickly and perfectly. Pinel, on the other hand, after many fruitless attempts, almost entirely gave up the practice amongst the old women at the Salpetriere. I believe that locality and social position exercise a deep but too frequently unregarded influence on the type of most inflammatory affections, and that while the inhabitant of the country, exposed to all the invigorating influences of nature, and leading a life more in accordance with her dictates, can well and advantageously bear the loss of blood, such a course is replete with peril in constitutions prematurely worn out by the pernicious habits of life that seem engendered in great cities. If the physician after carefully weighing all the circumstances of the case resolves on venesection, he must not postpone the operation. It is only at the very commencement of the attack that it can be serviceable; he must further bear in mind the slight reparative power of old age, and the fallacy of the pulse as an index of the propriety of prolonging or repeating venesection; nor must he overlook the fact that not unfrequently a slight depletion prescribed by men well qualified to judge of its fitness has been followed by increased oppression and collapse.

For my own part, I freely confess my extreme objection to general venesection in such cases. There is no evidence to show that in adult life venesection lessens the fatality of the disease; there is abundant evidence to show the danger of bleeding in old age, whether in a state of comparative health or disease.

Local depletions, either by leeches or cupping, are safer, and more manageable, than general venesection, and are, I firmly believe, with perhaps some very rare exceptions, equally serviceable in attacking the disease. As soon as there are indications of hepatization or suppuration, depletion must no longer be contemplated. When the bronchi begin to be filled with mucus, venesection would only tend to hasten the fatal result by lowering the forces, and thus offering an additional impediment to free expectoration; in short it would, or at all events might, give rise to suffocation.

As a general rule then, blood-letting, in any form, is only applicable in the early stage. Foremost amongst internal remedies we must place antimonials; but in old age as in childhood, they must be given with caution. Tartarized antimony is sometimes too depressing in its effects to be safely borne, and occasionally it is found, even in very small doses, to give rise to unmanageable diarrhœa. In these cases other preparations, as the white oxide of antimony (Ph. Ed.), the prepared sulphuret (Ph. Dub.), or the oxysulphuret may be given with advantage. I have often seen good results from the combination of slightly nauseating doses of antimony, or of ipecacuanha, with stimulating expectorants, such as squill or senega, in those cases in which there is a want of power to throw off the mucus from the bronchial tubes. In these instances camphor may be prescribed with advantage; it may be taken in doses of 2—5 grains every four hours, and may be combined with various other drugs, as for instance with antimony, if the inflammation approaches towards a sthenic character, or with musk, or a gum-resin, when the opposite character predominates. When the patient's strength is sufficiently great, a dose of ipecacuanha, sufficient to act as an emetic, will often afford striking relief. External irritants are valuable auxiliaries to internal remedies in these cases, especially where the vital powers are much depressed. Sinapisms to the legs are often useful; in cases in which the pneumonia seems connected with retrocedent gout, they should be continued to be applied at short intervals till the pain returns to the part originally affected. If the pneumonia assume from the commencement a very asthenic form, a large blister may be at once applied to the thorax, but should be removed as soon as there are any signs of vesication. With the same object in view I have often used blistering fluids, which are cleaner and less annoying to the patient, and at the same time equally serviceable. With similar objects in view, Copland strongly recommends the application of oil of turpentine, or of an embrocation consisting of equal parts of the compound camphor liniment, and of the turpentine liniment, with a little cajeput oil.

Of Purgatives I need say nothing; we must judge of their expediency by individual symptoms. Calomel and opium are no longer of the same use in the second stage that they were in earlier life; I think that at this period I have given muriate of ammonia with good effect; I have, at all events, seen patients rapidly improve under its use. Mercurial inunctions have been highly spoken of, but I have no experience of their effects.

In the third stage our main object is to support the patient's strength; there is no period at which he requires more constant attention: diffusible stimuli and vegetable tonics, wine, and strong beef-tea, form the principal remedies on which we can then base our slender hopes.

The diet must not be so rigorously antiphlogistic as in earlier life; it is seldom that we need place a positive interdict on weak chicken or mutton broths, or on jellies. Barley-water or toast and water may be allowed *ad libitum*.

The physician should never fail to warn his patient that an attack of pneumonia strongly predisposes to subsequent attacks, and should point out to him the increased danger of exposure to any causes, as chills, heats, neglect of colds, &c., that may prove injurious to the respiratory organs. He should also constantly bear in mind the fact to which I have already alluded, that in old persons the ordinary symptoms of pneumonia are often absent, or are so obscure as to escape common observation. This circumstance is dependent on the isolation, or the absence of sympathy between the different organs, which is noticed at some length in an early part of this volume. The following case, abridged from Grisolle, affords a striking illustration of the form of disease to which I refer. In the month of May he prescribed a laxative for an old woman at the Salpetriere, who had complained for some days previously of loss of appetite. She did not appear to be suffering from any severe disease and did not complain of any pain. The skin was not too hot; the pulse was rather frequent and irregular, but this was attributed to old disease of the heart. She took her meals, and walked about as usual during the day, but in the evening laid down and died suddenly. Fully persuaded that her death arose either from rupture of a vessel or softening of the brain, he was astonished to find no important morbid change, except gray hepatization of more than half the right lung. Similar cases have been recorded by Dalmas, and Hourmann and Dechambre. The last-named observers regard latent pneumonia as one of the causes of the sudden deaths which are so frequent in the asylums and hospitals for the aged.

SECTION II.

Bronchitis—Its Symptoms—Seat of Pain—Character of the Respiration—Expectoration—Venous Congestion—Fever—Causes—Progress—Prognosis—Treatment.

SENILE bronchitis is a disease of which the early *symptoms* are usually not very well marked. Occasionally there is a little cough, slight tightness of the chest, a general feeling of discomfort, and a sensation of weakness about the limbs. The patient soon complains of a burning feeling, most intense at the upper part of the sternum, and either extending towards the sides, or going downwards to the epigastric region. Sometimes the pain extends over the whole chest; it is not, however, so severe and cutting as in pneumonia. The respiration becomes difficult and gasping, and in a great measure abdominal; being most laboured during the evening and night, and compelling the patient to assume a partially upright position. A loud rhonchus is often perceptible both to the patient himself and the bystanders. The act of expectoration is very painful and straining, and only ejects a small quantity of tough, viscid, semi-opaque, grayish mucus, swimming in an abundance of serous fluid. A considerable quantity of this puriform matter is frequently ejected from the very commencement of the disease, without affording any relief to the patient. On listening to the chest with the stethoscope, or directly with the ear, we hear all sorts of mucous rhonchi, which are especially strong and large between the scapulæ and near the top of the sternum. The sound on percussion is comparatively dull, but not to be compared to that in pneumonia.

The state of the respiratory organs induces venous congestion, the effects of which are often shown, to a terrible degree, in the brain: the headache is sometimes excruciating, the jar caused by each cough making the head feel as if it were almost splitting. The lips and tongue, and often the whole face, present a livid appearance.

The fever is generally only slight; at first there are alternating shivering and hot fits, but after a time the latter condition becomes persistent, although at the same time the extremities are often cold, and the tips of the fingers blue. The pulse is accelerated, and is seldom hard, but is usually remarkable for its singular smallness. The fever and the local symptoms undergo an exacerbation as the evening advances.

Predisposing and exciting causes.—As a general rule, women are more frequently attacked than men, and a leucophlegmatic temperament seems especially to predispose towards this disease. Amongst the more specific predisposing causes we may arrange habits of intemperance, abdominal congestion, prolonged catarrhs and asthma, and the suppression of any habitual secretion. As is the case with most chest affections, the time of year and the state of the weather exert a considerable influence on the development of this disease. In cold, damp weather it sometimes appears quit e sporadic.

This disease is often very rapid in its *progress*, frequently terminating fatally in less than two days; its most common duration is a week or ten days. The not unfrequent cases of weak old people comparatively well, dying choaked with mucus before any assistance can arrive (the suffocative catarrh of Laennec), ought, I believe, to be placed under this head.

As the disease progresses to a favourable termination, the sputum becomes thicker, and assumes a yellow or greenish tint; the act of expectorating becomes easier, the respiration less laborious and the head freer. Any secretion that the disease may have checked is also restored to its ordinary state.

The *prognosis* is very unfavourable. The following are the principal grounds on which we must base it. (1) On the cause of the disease; bronchitis arising from cold is far less dangerous than when arising from the suppression of an ordinary secretion. (2) On the rapidity of the disease, the danger being proportional to the quickness of its progress. (3) On the topical symptoms—the characters of the respiration, sputa and voice, and the extent of venous congestion. (4) On the degree of febrile excitement. (5) On any complications that may occur in the course of the disease; pneumonia, pleurisy, or effusion into the pleura or pericardium, augments to a great degree the danger of the patient.

The leading indications in the *treatment* of bronchitis are to remove the pulmonary congestion and to free the bronchial tubes from the accumulation of mucus. The former point is best attained by depletion. We may occasionally meet with cases in which, during the early stage of the disease, six or eight ounces of blood may advantageously be taken from the arm, but as I have already remarked, great caution is requisite in prescribing venesection for aged people. To justify this treatment, the constitution of the patient should be moderately strong, the oppression at the chest very great, the respiration laboured, and the cough tearing and exhausting. Patients who would not bear venesection may often be cupped with great advantage.

Emetics in full doses are of much service in clearing out the loaded air passages. I have employed sulphate of zinc with much service in these cases, as being less depressing and less liable to irritate the bowels than tartar emetic, and less injurious to the system, if retained on the stomach, than sulphate of copper. After the emetic has freely acted, the expectoration must be kept up by slightly nauseating doses of ipecacuanha, antimonials, or squills; if there is much fever the former preparations are indicated; if the asthenic character predominates, squills, or a stimulating expectorant, as benzoic acid, may be given alone or in combination with ipecacuanha. Great advantage is often derived from the administration of camphor in this disease, and my own experience fully bears out the testimony of Dr. Copland, that when combined with colchicum, or with antimony, nitrate of potash, ipecacuanha, &c., and given in small doses in the more inflammatory and febrile states of the disease; when prescribed in progressively larger quantities with diuretics, the spirit. ether. nitr., opium, &c., as the vascular excitement subsides, and the febrile heat disappears; and in larger doses (from an ounce and a half to three ounces of Murray's solution), with ammonia, ammoniacum, senega, opium, &c., when exhaustion and difficulty of expectoration from deficient power are urgent, it is one of the most valuable remedies we possess.

When the febrile symptoms have nearly disappeared and the skin has become cool and moist, a large blister, or the frequent application of hot oil of turpentine, is often serviceable in preventing the fresh accumulation of mucus. If the vital powers are much depressed, the action of the blister may be aided by previously rubbing the skin with vinegar. It is of more importance to keep the bowels open in bronchitis than in pneumonia. The inhalation of medicated vapours is occasionally of great service in these cases. Much judgment is however required in their choice. In the early stages the vapour from emollient decoctions is most suitable. When the expectoration becomes opaque and thick, we may add a little strong vinegar, or camphor, or tincture of hyoscyamus to the decoction; and if the disease assumes a very asthenic character we may recommend the inhalation of much more stimulating vapours, as those of tar, the balsams, and even chlorine very much diluted with atmospheric air. Much harm has resulted from the application of medicated vapours in too concentrated a state; and this has doubtless been the reason why this mode of treatment has never been generally adopted.

With respect to diet, it must be mildly antiphlogistic. Weak broths and jellies may usually be allowed, with the free use of barley-water and toast and water. The temperature of the patient's room should be carefully looked to, and I may take this opportunity of directing attention to the degree of moisture in the sick room. A fire in a closed room dries the air, which the patient has to breathe, to such a degree as to irritate the bronchial mucous membrane. The dry and wet bulb thermometer is here of the greatest value in enabling us to judge of the humidity of the atmosphere in the apartment. If the air be too dry or the difference between the readings of the two thermometers be too great, it will be necessary to expose water in a shallow vessel of some extent of surface, so that the vapour from the water will mix with the air and moisten it; if this be required to be done quickly, the water may be heated and then exposed, and the evaporation will go on more quickly; the reading of the wet bulb will point out when the proper degree of humidity is attained; in the case of heated water, it may then be removed, in the case of cold water, it may be allowed to remain; and if it be found that the air is becoming too damp, a smaller surface of water may be exposed, which surface may be increased, should it be found that the air does not remain sufficiently damp.

The instrument must be placed in a part of the room away from the fire, so that no straight line can be drawn from the fire to it, and it must not be exposed to open doors or currents of air.

A difference of about 10° between the readings of the two thermometers will generally be found to give a pleasant degree of humidity to persons in a state of health.* In bronchitis, and indeed in most diseases of the respiratory organs, a greater degree of humidity, indicated by a smaller difference between the wet and dry bulb thermometers, affords more relief to the patient; and this is a point on which he may be safely allowed to judge for himself.

The bronchitis of old people frequently terminates in a chronic secretion of mucus, resulting from want of tone in the mucous membrane. This must be combated by the balsams, gum-resins, and astringents. Amongst the medicines in most repute we may mention the decoction of Iceland moss, the balsams of tolu and copaiva, guaiacum, quinine, the compound tincture of bark, and the mineral acids. They must be administered (with the exception of the Iceland moss) in small doses, for if the secretion is too rapidly checked, the most serious consequences may ensue. A moderate allowance of wine and a strengthening diet should also then be prescribed.

SECTION III.

Chronic Bronchorrhœa, or the Mucous Flux of the Aged—Its Symptoms—Causes—Progress—Connexion with other Diseases—Prognosis—Treatment.

A MODERATE amount of mucous expectoration, accompanied with cough, is so common in old persons, especially on first waking, that it may be regarded as the rule rather than the exception. The expectorated matter is tough, thick, and of a pale yellow or yellowish-

---

* For an excellent account of this instrument, and its various applications, I may refer to Mr. Glaisher's *Hygrometrical Tables*. 1847.

green tint; it is brought up without the least exertion on the part of the patient, and it becomes such a matter of course with him, that at length he altogether ceases to regard it. The amount of bronchial secretion may, however, increase to a very serious degree. It may amount to many ounces in the course of the day; and simultaneously with this augmentation we hear complaints of shortness of breath, of tightness or fulness of the chest, and of a sensation of pressure on the upper part of the centre of the chest. On further inquiry we find that this shortness of breath is increased to a painful extent on going up stairs, and that the patient is most at his ease when the head and chest are kept in a somewhat elevated position. The *symptoms* are aggravated by sudden atmospheric vicissitudes, especially by the change from moist to dry weather, and by the suppression of any ordinary discharges, as for instance by sudden attacks of constipation, or by the stoppage of leucorrhœa in the female.

With the exception of the symptoms we have already mentioned, the chest is free from pain; it can be expanded to its full extent at will, and the patient can rest equally well on either side.

On auscultation, the respiratory manner is found to be weak, and to be mixed with more or less sibilous rhonchus; and evidences of bronchial dilatation are not unfrequently afforded. The sounds elicited by percussion are usually normal.

The general symptoms are usually very trifling, excepting in those cases where the tendency to the secretion of mucus propagates itself to the other mucous tracts—to the digestive and the urinary organs.

When the bronchial secretion is very abundant, its derivative influence becomes apparent on the ordinary normal secretions: the skin becomes dry and scaly, the bowels become constipated, and the amount of urine is much diminished. If the disease proceeds unchecked, evening febrile exacerbations usually ensue, and the patient finally sinks from emaciation and exhaustion.

The female sex is more liable to this affection than the male. Amongst other predisposing *causes*, we may mention an atonic state of the constitution, numerous antecedent catarrhal attacks, the general influence of certain trades which require a continuous exposure to a moist and impure atmosphere, and a residence in a low marshy country.

But independently of external causes, attacks of bronchorrhœa may often be traced to various internal sources of irritation. As bronchorrhœa occasionally gives rise to derangement of the digestive and urinary organs, so the converse also holds good. There is often a very close association between this affection and gout, piles, suppression of urine, checked perspiration, or the too rapid cure of ulcers, issues, or discharging skin-diseases.

The *progress* of bronchorrhœa is usually very slow; it is a disease that may go on for very many years. In moist wintry weather it is at its worst; in the dry warmth of summer the patient has a temporary respite; for two or three months, or longer in a more genial atmosphere than ours, he may almost forget that he is an invalid, and may delude himself into the idea that his enemy has departed from him. The first blast of winter will undeceive him. And so he goes on from year to year. The disease is too often structural and incurable; and well it is for the sufferer if it only remains stationary. When it is connected with gout or suppression of the secretions, we not very unfrequently have an alternation of disease; a paroxysm of gout, or an increased discharge of urine or sweat, will often wonderfully relieve the pulmonary affection.

In establishing our *prognosis* we must be guided by the following points:—

1. The age of the patient: the older he is, the less able will he be to cope with the disease.

2. The length of his illness.

3. Whether he has been in the habit of suffering from catarrhal affections, this being an unfavourable symptom.

4. The character of the expectoration. If it continues to increase in quantity, assumes a purulent appearance, and evolves a fœtid odour, we are led to augur badly for our patient.

5. We must be guided by the general symptoms,—the state of the respiration, the mode in which the cutaneous and urinary functions are discharged, and the presence or absence of emaciation and fever. Concomitant disease of the heart, or dropsy, greatly increases the danger.

The leading indications with regard to the *treatment* of this disease are, first, to remove, if possible, the exciting cause; and, secondly, to give increased tonicity to the bronchial mucous membrane.

1. Nothing is so generally effectual in checking this disease as a removal to a dry warm climate. When this remedy is beyond the patient's means, as is too often the case, he should be recommended to confine himself to a suite of rooms kept at a constant and rather

high temperature; and if the weather should be moist and foggy, it may be advisable that vessels containing chloride of calcium or strong sulphuric acid should be placed in the apartments. All exposure to morning and evening chills, even in the finest climate, must be carefully avoided, and this remark applies even more forcibly to running the chance of getting wet.

The clothing should be warm; and flannel, or what are termed union-dresses, should be worn next the skin.

The diet should contain a fair proportion of easily digestible animal food; the dinner hour should not be later than three or four o'clock, and nothing should be taken for at least a couple of hours before retiring to rest. Good well-hopped beer and a couple of glasses of port* may generally be taken with advantage. Passive exercise, as sailing or driving, may always be allowed in dry, warm weather.

The cutaneous system requires special attention in these cases: the flesh-brush should be vigorously used by an attendant night and morning, and we often find it advisable to excite the skin by irritating baths or lotions.

If the disease is connected with the suppression of any secretion, no attempt should be omitted to overcome that suppression. If ulcers on the legs or feet have been recently healed, an open blister should be kept in their vicinity, or the ulcers themselves allowed to reappear. If abdominal plethora be suspected to be the cause, gentle aperients and a subsequent course of appropriate mineral waters are usually serviceable. Previous to the removal or diminution of the source of irritation, we must not expect to derive any advantage from the use of tonics and astringents.

2. In carrying out the second stage of treatment we must be careful not to suppress the mucous discharge too suddenly. Without attending to this precaution, we might induce bronchial paralysis and suffocation. It is advisable to commence with a dose of ipecacuanha, sufficiently large to act as an emetic. This clears the bronchi and stomach of a large quantity of viscid mucus, and thus prepares the system for the action of strengthening medicines. As I have mentioned in an early part of this volume, we should always endeavour to select our tonics from the vegetable kingdom. We have a copious field to choose from. Cinchona and its various preparations,

* I prefer port in these cases, in consequence of its astringent properties.

cascarilla, quassia, marrubium, &c., should be combined with aromatics and expectorants—with small doses of ipecacuanha, antimony, or squills, and of sulphur or some aromatic stimulant. When these medicines begin to lose their effect, we may safely proceed to the more powerful astringents—to the mineral acids, balsams, creosote, myrrh, kino, catechu, and turpentine. The inhalation of the diluted vapours of chlorine, tar, and the different balsams and gum-resins is often extremely serviceable ; if, however, they give rise to pulmonary irritation, their use must be immediately suspended. We can often relieve the bronchial membrane by the application of revulsives and derivatives. Common vapour or sulphur baths, turpentine or other stimulating embrocations, dry cupping, purgatives, and diuretics, all act in this manner. When the patient is of a gouty habit, small doses of colchicum usually afford singular relief.

I have sometimes found great service from a very mild mercurial treatment in these cases. A grain of blue pill, an eighth of a grain of tartar emetic, and two or three grains of extract of conium forms a good combination in these cases, and may be taken three times a-day, for four or five days, then twice a-day for an equal time, and finally once a-day for a week.

When bronchorrhœa is associated with asthma, antispasmodics may be freely administered. (See the following Section.)

SECTION IV.

Asthma—A Symptom rather than a Disease—Different Forms of Asthma— General Principles of Treatment.

I have already taken occasion to remark that it is not my object in this volume to write histories of disease. I have treated of some diseases fully, either because I conceive they had hitherto not met with the consideration they demanded, or because the differences they presented in early and advanced life were especially striking.

With asthma neither reason holds good ; although the number of deaths of aged persons ascribed to it is very considerable, I suspect that in most instances its primary attack has been made during the period of mature life. It is an essentially chronic affection, killing as it were by small instalments. Out of the 51,048 deaths at or about the age of 60, occurring in London during the five years extending from the commencement of 1843 to that of 1848, no less than 3,312 are ascribed to asthma. I likewise find that the number of deaths from this disease occurring at or above the age of 60 is nearly double that of the whole of the earlier period of life. In 1847 the deaths at and above 60 were 793, whilst those under that age were 426, or little more than half that number.

Asthma is a disorder on the description of which much unnecessary refinement has been practised.* I trust that in these pages I have succeeded in clearing up some of the obscurities with which medical writers have contrived to envelop the true nature of the affection.

By asthma I mean *an intermittent difficulty of breathing*. It is not strictly speaking a disease so much as a symptom of various morbid conditions of the system. It is associated with certain states of the bronchial tubes, with emphysema and œdema of the lungs, with hypertrophy and dilatation of the heart, with valvular disease, and with dilatation of the arch of the aorta. It is difficult in many cases to decide which is the primary and which the secondary affection. This I term *organic asthma*.

Another form, almost precisely similar in its manifestations, is dependent on an impure condition of the blood; it chiefly occurs in persons of a gouty habit, or in whom the action of the kidneys is torpid. It is this form of the disease which occasionally follows the too rapid cure of a discharging cutaneous eruption, of an ulcer, or any other drain upon the system. For want of a better term we may name it *cachectic asthma* or *asthma from an impure condition of the blood*. I very much doubt whether the form termed *pure nervous asthma*, ever occurs in advanced life. As far as my personal experience goes I have never had any difficulty, after a careful examination of the thoracic organs in the intervals between the paroxysms, and a full inquiry regarding the previous health of the patient, in placing every case that has come before me under one of the two former heads.

Asthma is described as *dry* or as *humid*, according to the degree of expectoration that occurs towards the close of the paroxysm.

In the chronic bronchorrhœa of old persons (see Section III.), especially when a fresh attack is engrafted on a former one, so great and sudden an increase of mucus often takes place as to close some

* Sauvages has enumerated eighteen forms of this disease. Dr. Mason Good divided this disease into the *dry* and the *humid,* subdividing these forms into eight varieties.

of the larger bronchial tubes, and prevent the passage of air through them. The habitual difficulty of breathing becomes suddenly increased, and the patient is only relieved by a free expectoration of mucus, after which he returns to his former state.

The premonitory *symptoms* are occasionally so distinct as to enable the physician to foretell the advent of paroxysm with tolerable certainty. Drowsiness is a common symptom; eructations, flatulent distention of the stomach, and the general symptoms of dyspepsia are also usually observed for a day or two before the attack.

This species of asthma usually comes on soon after the patient is in bed, and the accumulation of mucus on which the paroxysm depends seems partly due to the change of position. Fits of asthma from this cause are generally renewed every four or five days if the weather be cold and damp, and are seldom altogether got rid of, till the atmosphere becomes warm and genial. In very debilitated persons we often find that the power of expectorating is so much diminished, that the secretion cannot be ejected. I need hardly point out the necessary consequences of this inability: the dyspnœa increases, the face becomes ghastly and livid, partial coma supervenes from the absence of duly aerated blood, and the patient dies suffocated.

Dry asthma is associated with emphysema of the lungs, but on this form of asthma, and on that from cardiac disease, I have no remarks to offer, except in relation to treatment.

I proceed to the subject of *cachectic asthma*—an affection that seems to have been almost altogether overlooked by English practitioners, although of very common occurrence. The impurities contained in the blood seem here to be the exciting cause of the paroxysm. There is an attempt on the part of nature to make the bronchial mucous membrane eliminate the effete matter of the blood in the form of expectoration.

Asthma is very often associated with a deficient or morbid action of the kidneys. I have seen so many cases of this form of asthma that I cannot doubt the intimate connection between the state of the respiration and the morbid condition of the kidney, and for the sake of convenience shall term this *urinous asthma*. The term has been already used by Schonlein, Canstatt, and other continental writers, therefore I do not incur the charge of introducing a new name into our medical nomenclature.

The following are the most important points in reference to urinous asthma. It seldom occurs before the 60th year, and is most common at and beyond the 70th year. On examining a patient with this affection we usually find a general suppression of the secretions, the skin being dry and rough, and the bowels acting slightly about twice a week. The urine is scanty, rather turbid, of a reddish-brown colour, and so acrid as to produce a sensation of scalding in the urethra, and to give rise to frequent calls to make water. There is usually a feeling of dull, deep-seated pain about the loins. The skin is the seat of intolerable itching, and presents the appearance of prurigo, which, like the asthma, arises from the retention of the urinary constituents in the blood. The eyelids are red, and discharge an acrid humour; and ulcers often form on the lower extremities. These are evidences of the striving of the system to throw off the morbid matter accumulated in the blood; they are, however, not sufficient for the proposed end, and the bronchial mucous membrane is called upon to aid in the work of purification. Such are the conditions giving rise to this form of asthma, and it is worthy of notice, that it seems often to alternate with the other unpleasant symptoms of deficient renal action—as for instance, with prurigo, ulcers on the legs, and the peculiar kind of conjunctivitis to which I have just alluded. The paroxysm usually occurs an hour or two before midnight, and lasts some hours, terminating most commonly in a copious expectoration of viscid and very salt mucus, which frequently has a strong, urinous odour; at the same time a copious perspiration breaks out over the chest. In patients with this form of asthma there is seldom a perfect remission, there being almost invariably a certain degree of tightness of the chest and of shortness of breath.

Another cachectic form of asthma is connected with the gouty diathesis. It sometimes comes on as early as the 50th year in persons suffering from asthenic or anomalous gout. The premonitory symptoms are the same as those of a fit of regular gout. There are complaints of general discomfort, tightness and weight in the precordia, loss of appetite, flatulence, acid eructations and vomitings, and sometimes a tingling sensation about the parts which have been the previous seat of gout.

The patient is led by these symptoms to expect a fit of gout; but instead of this, he is seized, usually about midnight or a little before, with a feeling of intense and terrible suffocation. The face assumes a livid appearance, and is generally swollen, the jugular veins are tense and fully distended, mucus tinged with blood dribbles from the lips, and the heart's action is weak and intermittent; the paroxysm lasts, with slight remissions, for some hours, and towards its close a considerable amount of thick mucus, frequently mixed with blood, is ejected. The fit is often succeeded by other efforts to depurate the system—by copious sweats, urinary sediments, &c. If they do not occur, a second paroxysm of asthma may be very shortly expected. This form of asthma is in short neither more nor less than misplaced gout.

These illustrations are sufficient to elucidate my views regarding the two great forms of asthma.

In the treatment of asthma, it is most essential to distinguish the cause on which it depends; this, however, is often a task of considerable difficulty. The humid asthma depending on bronchorrhœa is best treated during the intervals by tonics combined with expectorants. When the attack is felt to be coming on, an emetic is often highly serviceable; mustard poultices should be applied over the chest and pit of the stomach, and the feet and legs placed in hot water. Musk is a valuable remedy in these cases, and deserves a more general trial than it has yet received from the profession.

Asthma, connected with other morbid states of the respiratory organs, is best treated by keeping the skin in a state of activity, by the frequent application of counter-irritants, and by establishing artificial discharges by means of tartar-emetic ointment, croton oil, or even a seton. The action of the bowels must be aided by gentle aperients, and the kidneys should be stimulated to an increased action. The administration of the fetid gum resins, of squill, or of small doses of antimony serves to increase the bronchial secretion, and thus relieve the congested state of the bronchial mucous membrane. The violence of the spasmodic action that is more or less present in all asthmatic attacks, whatever be the cause from which they arise, must be opposed by sedative and antispasmodic remedies. Musk, camphor, valerianate of zinc, the lobelia inflata, and stramonium are here applicable; strong coffee has also been much recommended.

The calmative effect of stramonium in many cases of asthma is perfectly astonishing. The following is the way in which I generally advise it to be taken. If the patient is a tobacco smoker, I order 15 or 20 grains of dried stramonium leaves to be mixed with enough tobacco to fill the pipe. If he has fortunately not indulged in that pernicious but too common habit, I substitute dried sage leaves for tobacco. Women are not so liable to asthma as men; in their case, if they cannot be prevailed upon to try this form of treatment, we must throw the leaves on a chafing dish of hot coals or on a heated iron plate, and allow the vapour to diffuse itself through the apartment.

Cigarettes made according to the following prescription have been extensively used on the Continent, and doubtless present a useful combination.

Take Picked leaves of Belladonna	6 grains
Hyoscyamus	
Stramonium, each	3 grains
Phellandrium aquaticum	1 grain
Aqueous extract of Opium	¼ of a grain
Cherry-laurel water	a sufficiency.

The leaves must have the nerves removed previously to chopping and mixing them; the opium must be dissolved in the cherry-laurel water, and diffused through the mass. From two to four of these cigarettes may be smoked by asthmatic persons, when they apprehend or are seized with a paroxysm.

In the treatment of asthma arising from a diminished secretion of urine, our great aim must be to obtain a proper action of the kidneys. I have several times observed that diuretics were of little service until a few ounces of blood had been taken from the loins. Occasionally we find that even after the abstraction of a little blood, the kidneys fail to be excited to increased action by diuretics. We must then act as powerfully as we can on the skin, by hot baths, vapour baths, &c. We must be especially careful in such cases not to heal any ulcers, or discharging skin-diseases, which are then acting as outlets for the noxious matter of the blood.

The treatment of gouty asthma is much the same as that for other forms of misplaced gout, and is described in Chapter XIII.

I will conclude these miscellaneous observations on asthma with a few remarks which are equally applicable to every form of it. I never met with an asthmatic old person who was not subject to dyspepsia. Hence close attention to the stomach and bowels is requisite. The warmer purgatives combined with antacids are most serviceable in these cases. Ten or twelve grains of Gregory's powder, or a combination of rhubarb with carbonate of soda and calumba, should be taken regularly for ten days or a fortnight, whenever dyspeptic symptoms begin to show themselves. It may be taken either before dinner or at bedtime in a wine-glassful of water, or wine and water. The diet should be light, but at the same time nutritious. All indigestible food should be carefully avoided, and the stomach should never be filled to repletion. In fact the dietetic treatment must be precisely the same as in cases of simple dyspepsia. The chest should be daily washed with cold water, containing a handful of salt or a little vinegar, and rubbed till a genial glow is produced. The clothing had better be too warm than too cold, and especial care should be taken to protect the feet from cold or wet. An asthmatic person should never expose himself to sudden changes of temperature, and should religiously eschew theatres, ball-rooms, and all crowded and over-heated places, with an atmosphere poisoned by the exhalations of his brother-mortals.

SECTION V.

HYDROTHORAX AND PULMONARY ŒDEMA.

HYDROTHORAX is scarcely ever (I believe I may say, never) a primary affection in advanced life.

It arises either:

1. From certain organic changes in the lungs, heart, or larger vessels, from extreme ossification of the cartilages of the ribs, from morbid deposits on the pleura, &c. Hence its frequent association with asthma, the paroxysms of which doubtless favour the process of effusion into the pleural cavity, by the venous congestion to which they give rise.

2. Or from metastatic action connected (α) with gout (β), with too rapidly healed ulcers on the legs or feet, or (γ) with the sudden stoppage of the bronchial flux.

Collections of fluid arising from organic changes, accumulate very slowly, and the symptoms often escape the notice both of the patient and the physician for some time. When however they depend on the sudden retrogression of gout or other analogous causes, their progress is often very rapid.

I shall confine my remarks on this affection to a few observations on treatment.

It is seldom that in cases of hydrothorax in persons of advanced life we can hope for a perfect cure. The first and most important point is to ascertain the cause of the effusion; but at the same time we must do all in our power to alleviate the dyspnœa and other distressing symptoms produced by the fluid in the pleural sac. For this second point our treatment must be much the same as that recommended in asthma.

When the effusion is connected with cardiac disease, considerable service is sometimes derived from the insertion of a seton over the region of the heart. We must simultaneously endeavour to increase the secretion of the bronchial mucous membrane.

When it arises from retrocedent gout or the sudden cure of an old ulcer, we must endeavour in the one case to recall the gout to the extremities, and in the other we must establish a discharge by a seton or blisters at or near the site of the ulcer.

With regard to the removal of the effused fluid our means are unfortunately very limited. Drastic purgatives by their depressing effect on the system are more likely to do harm than good. Diuretics are however often very serviceable in these cases. Of this class of medicines digitalis is the most valuable; and its efficacy seems to be increased by combining with it small quantities of blue pill or calomel, and opium. Camphor may also be very advantageously associated with it. These remedies failing us, we may try squills, the diuretic salts, colchicum, infusion of buchu with compound spirit of juniper, and other remedies tending to augment the urinary secretion.

I doubt whether in these cases paracentesis is ever advisable.

I place œdema of the lungs in the same section with hydrothorax. It arises from much the same causes, presents very nearly the same symptoms, and requires very similar treatment. Dropsy of the pericardium is often associated with these affections.

SECTION VI.

PULMONARY CONSUMPTION AND HÆMOPTYSIS.

The only reason for my making a passing allusion to pulmonary consumption is in consequence of the considerable number of deaths described in the Mortality Tables as occurring from it, at or after the age of 60.* In the majority of these cases the seeds of the disease

* Of 53,048 deaths at or above the age of 60, 1867 are ascribed to this disease. Out of 122 cases of recent and well-marked tubercular disease of the lungs, Hasse

were doubtless sown at an earlier period of life; but there are instances—and they constitute a very respectable minority—in which this affection first develops itself and runs a very rapid course in advanced life.

The following case will serve to illustrate the former point:—

Case of protracted phthisis.—In the month of December, 1834, Dr. Morton, of Philadelphia, was requested to see Mrs. S. T. She was an extremely thin and delicate person, with very dark hair and sallow complexion. She was 64 years of age, was the mother of eleven children, and had suffered with pain in the left side (chiefly beneath the clavicle and in the axillary region), with cough and occasional fever, for forty-five years. Twenty-four years ago, she had an attack of hæmoptysis, consisting of florid, frothy blood, in considerable quantity. The cough and fever from that time became, and have continued much worse, and were liable to aggravation by every change of weather. During twenty-three of the above twenty-five years she was accustomed to use great bodily exertion, without regard to weather, often exposing herself to cold, wet, and fatigue, in a rigorous climate. During the two last years (from 1832 to 1834), she has resided in Philadelphia, has been much less active, and much more complaining. "Her expectoration," says Dr. Morton, in December, 1834, "is decidedly purulent, and her fever hectic. On applying the stethoscope I readily detected a small abscess beneath the apex of the left lung, around which spot, to a great distance, the respiration was extremely defective. The upper lobe of the right

observed that fourteen preceded the 20th, seventy-four intervened between the 20th and 40th, twenty-six between the 40th and 60th, seven between the 60th and 80th, and one occurred subsequently to the 80th year. In 100 cases, above the age of 15, Bayle found that fifteen occurred between the ages of 50 and 60, and eight between 60 and 70. In 123 cases (also above the age of 15) observed by Louis, twelve occurred between the ages of 50 and 60, and five between 60 and 70. Of 497 deaths from this disease in the Philadelphia Almshouse Hospital, the patients ranging from 18 upwards, there occurred—

From 18 to 35	. . . .	263
" 35 " 40	. . . .	73
" 40 " 50	. . . .	78
" 50 " 60	. . . .	47
" 60 " 70	. . . .	24
" 70 " 80	. . . .	8
" 80 " 90	. . . .	2
" 90 " 100	. . . .	2—See Morton's *Illustration of Pulmonary Consumption*, 2d edit. p. 70.

lung was almost equally defective, but gave no evidence of a cavity. In this example, habitual activity of body and mind has kept the malady at bay for a very long series of years; but as exercise gives place to indulgence, the disease assumes a more acute character, and makes more rapid progress.

"Two years afterwards (Dec. 1836), having suffered an exacerbation of disease during the last summer, she took a long journey to her former residence in Vermont, and came back much recruited; but inactivity has again reduced her strength, which she finds to be exactly in proportion to the exercise she uses in the open air.

"There is good reason to believe," adds Dr. Morton, "that in this instance tuberculous disease has continued for forty-seven years. How much of this time the abscess has been in the lung, is impossible to say; but the patient assures me that she has had, for twenty-seven years, the same expectoration, febricula, and slight but frequent hemoptysis, that she labours under at present, rendering it more than probable that her lung has been ulcerated during the whole of that long period."

Dr. Latham mentions cases in which persons were twelve and twenty years dying from this complaint. Hence there can be no doubt that in a larger number of the deaths at and after the age of sixty, the disease has been slowly progressing, or at all events existing for some time.

The case CXV. in Dr. Blakiston's Treatise on Diseases of the Chest, to which work I must refer my readers for particulars regarding it, shows, on the other hand, *how rapid the progress of the malady may be* even in advanced life.

It is that of a labourer aged seventy-three years, previously in good health, who died from acute pulmonary phthisis after an illness of only eight weeks.

The treatment of this disease, in advanced life, requires no peculiar notice. I trust, as in earlier life, to a combination of tonics and sedatives, and to counter-irritants. Amongst the tonics, I place the most confidence in cod-liver oil, and iodide of iron.

I have no remarks to offer on the symptoms, except to observe that we must not forget, in reference to auscultation and percussion, the modified condition of the lungs (see pages 29 and 72), and the altered sounds to which they give rise; and further to state my conviction that in advanced life, hæmoptysis, which in earlier life is so fearful a symptom, is here of comparatively little consequence.

In persons suffering from suppressed hæmorrhoids, the pulmonary veins seem to assume a varicose state, and relief is often afforded by the hæmoptysis. In these cases, if we cannot restore the hæmorrhoidal flux by irritant purgatives, we can often do so by injecting into the rectum an enema containing four or five grains of aloes, or a few drops of oil of savine in an emulsion. A few leeches applied to the anus often exert a strong derivative influence in these cases.

SECTION VII.

INFLUENZA.

Its Nature—Fatality—History of the Epidemic of 1847—Its Causes—Symptoms—Treatment.

ALTHOUGH influenza is a febrile disorder affecting the whole system, the catarrh is so marked a symptom that I have deemed it advisable to notice the disease in the present chapter.

The following remarks from the Registrar-General's Report *on the State of the Public Health in the last quarter of the year* 1847, are of such high interest, that I need offer no apology for extracting them.

"Influenza, like small-pox, probably always exists; in ordinary circumstances it is confounded with inflammation of the air-tubes, yet in London from one to five deaths have been directly referred to it, every week since the new London Tables were published. Like other zymotic* diseases it becomes at intervals of some years epidemic; that is, it attacks the people generally of all classes. Its epidemics are distinguished by the numbers they assail; by affecting the same person more than once; by being most fatal to the aged; by great differences in the severity and fatality of their attacks; by the rapidity of their course, and passage from place to place. After the mortality they occasion becomes apparent in London, it attains a maximum in the *second* or *third* week; and the mortality falls to the average in the *sixth or seventh* week. Influenza appears to be generated in ill-organized camps, and in crowded, ill-cleansed cities; and to be most fatal among people who have for some time been de-

---

* The term *zymotic* in the mortality tables embraces *endemic, epidemic,* and *infectious* diseases.

pressed, ill-fed, or ill-supplied with vegetables, as after hard winters and in war; it rages in cold and hot, moist and dry weather, but most frequently breaks out after a thaw, or with violence after a fog, generally the result of cold streams of air mixed with warm air—and a calm.

"The saturation of the atmosphere favours the transportation of all organic matters; and those of a zymotic character among the rest. Extreme cold only, never raises the weekly mortality in London above 1500; extreme heat still less; intermediate changes affect the mortality but slightly in ordinary circumstances; November fogs occur every year without giving rise to influenza; in November, 1847, the weather was nearly the same all over England, yet influenza did not break out simultaneously. When once generated the epidemic spreads through the air. The great epidemics generally travel from (1) Russia, over (2) Germany, (3) Denmark, Sweden, England, France, (4) Italy, Spain, in from three to six months; and then reach America. Influenza is often associated with other epidemics. It appears to have preceded or accompanied the plague in the black death of the fourteenth century; it preceded the great plague of London (1665); it followed epidemic typhus in London, 1803, preceded it in 1837; occurred in the midst of the typhus epidemic of 1847; preceded and followed the epidemic cholera in 1831-2-3. It carries off asthmatic persons, and those suffering from chronic diseases; it affects those labouring under other zymotic diseases; in the healthy it quickens the seeds of other maladies, particularly of the lungs.

"The fatality and duration of its attacks vary with age. In some of the late epidemics two in one hundred cases attended by medical men are said to have died; if this was the rate of mortality for London, for 5000 deaths, there must have been 250,000 cases of sickness of not less than seven days' duration. This would be little more than one in eight of the population; but nearly all were affected more or less, and without taking slight instances it is probable that not less than 500,000 persons in 2,100,000 suffered in London from the epidemic of 1847."

The epidemic of last year must be so fresh in the memory of my readers that the following observations regarding it will probably be read with interest. It is stated in the valuable report from which the above extract is taken, that although typhus and scarlatina were prevalent, the deaths registered in the metropolis in the last week of

October were only 945 (the weekly average during the autumn, as deduced from the four preceding years, being 1046); one person died of influenza, thirty-six of bronchitis, and sixty-two of pneumonia. In the three weeks following, ending November 20, the total deaths were 1052, 1098, and 1086, of which two, four, and four were by influenza; forty-nine, fifty-eight, and sixty-one were by bronchitis; sixty-eight, seventy-nine, and ninety-five by pneumonia. The wind had generally been blowing S.S.W. and S.W. since the first week of October; the weather was unusually warm; on Tuesday, November 16th, the wind changed to N.W., and amidst various changes blew from the north over Greenwich, at the rate of 160 to 250 miles a day. The mean temperature of the air suddenly fell from 11° above to 10° below the average; on Monday it was 54°, on Friday 32°; the air on Friday night was 27°; the earth was frozen; the wind was calm three days, and on Saturday evening a dense fog lay over London for five hours. No electricity stirred in the air during the week. All was still: as if Nature held her breath at the sight of the destroyer, come forth to sacrifice her children. On Sunday the sky was overcast, the air damp, the wind changed in the night to south by east, and passed for four days over Greenwich at the rate of 200 to 300 miles daily; the temperature suddenly rose, and remained from 2° to 9° above the average through the week ending November 27th, when the deaths of 1677 persons were registered, of which 338 were of the age of 60 and upwards. Influenza was epidemic. On the first week of December *two thousand, four hundred, and fifty-four* persons died, of whom 730 were of the age of 60 and upwards. On the week following *two thousand, four hundred and sixteen* died, of whom 702 were of the age of 60 and upwards. The deaths in the weeks ending Saturday, December 18, December 25, and January 1, were 1946, 1247, and 1599; 11,339 persons died in London in the space of six weeks, and altogether the epidemic carried off more than 5000 souls over and above the ordinary mortality of the season. It attained the greatest intensity in the second week of its course; raged with nearly equal violence through the third week; declined in the fourth, and then partly subsided.

The epidemic was most fatal to adults and to the aged. During a period of three weeks the mortality in childhood was raised eighty-three per cent., in manhood one hundred and four per cent., but in old age *two hundred and forty-seven* per cent.

Influenza attacked those labouring under all sorts of diseases as well as the healthy. The vital force was extinguished in old age and in persons suffering from chronic diseases. The poison permeating the whole system, fastened chiefly on the mucous membrane lining the sinuses of the face and head, and the air-tubes of the lungs. Hence it was fatal to the asthmatic; the deaths directly ascribed to asthma in October and November were twelve weekly; in the six weeks of the influenza epidemic 77, 86, 78, 52, 14, 26, besides the numerous cases classed under influenza. Thirty-six deaths were ascribed to bronchitis in the week ending October 30th, and 49, 58, 61, 196, 343, 299, 234, 107, and 138 in the nine weeks following. In some of these cases the inflammation specified was the primary disease, in others it was secondary, and in many it was purely influenza—mis-reported. The influence exerted by this disease on other zymotic diseases is well worthy of notice. Thus, the fatal cases of typhus, which were seventy or eighty, rose during the second, third, and fourth weeks of the influenza to 132, 136, 131.

We must say a word or two on the origin of influenza—a subject on which we unfortunately have no certain knowledge.

In addition to the oxygen, nitrogen, carbonic acid and aqueous vapour constituting the atmosphere, there is always a certain amount of organic matter in it. The chemist can recognise no difference in the composition of the air at the top of Mount Blanc and in the valley beneath it, through which perchance a hare, a fox, or a man has passed; but still the acute nose of the hound shows that a difference does exist. And so it is with the air which produces small-pox, measles, scarlatina, influenza, typhus, and plague; although the most subtle chemistry detects no peculiarity, we have fatal evidence that a peculiarity does exist. The emanations from the living and the dead, from the slaughter-houses, and the Thames foul with the produce of reeking sewers, raise over London an atmosphere of organic decomposing matter, and it is very possible that this matter differently modified by meteorological and other physical agents may at one time give rise to typhus, at another to influenza, and at a third perhaps to cholera.*

A theory has been recently propounded by an eminent German chemist (Schönbein, the discoverer of gun-cotton) that epidemic influenza is dependent on the presence of an imponderable agent termed *ozone*, in the atmosphere. This ozone is apparently a result of atmo-

* In the above remarks I have freely availed myself of the valuable report already alluded to.

spheric electricity. It may be prepared in the laboratory of the chemist, and from what we know of its properties there are à priori reasons for suspecting that it would, if existing in the air we breathe, give rise to great irritation of the respiratory organs. Several physicians have actually found that an excess of this material* was present in the atmosphere during the late epidemic.

With regard to the symptoms, it may be observed that although in minor points each epidemic presents its own peculiarities, there is great uniformity amongst those of a more important character.

The febrile symptoms commence with more or less rigor, pain in the back, and muscular pains generally. There is a feeling of great discomfort, prostration, and weariness of oneself and everybody besides, a feeling of great weight, and often of intense pain in the forehead and over the eyes. Soreness and tenderness of the throat are often complained of, and there is considerable hoarseness. Tightness and constriction of the chest, and soreness beneath the sternum are often remarked, patients complaining that they felt as if an iron band were pressed around the thorax. The muscular pains continue as at first. The eyes are injected and filled with tears; the nostrils are sore from the irritative character of their secretion; the tongue is covered with a white or yellow cream-like coating, but is usually of a bright red colour at the tip. The cough is one of the most distressing symptoms, often being so frequent as to prevent sleep, and almost always aggravating the headache. The expectoration presents no striking peculiarity; it generally is scanty at the commencement, and consists of merely a little clear viscid mucus, brought up with difficulty; as the disease progresses, it becomes more free and abundant,

---

* As every thing connected with the cause of epidemics is of extreme importance, I give the following simple method of determining whether there be an excess of ozone in the atmosphere. Ozone is a very intense oxidizing agent; and it is on this property that the following test is based. Every one knows that free iodine acting on starch gives rise to a beautiful blue colour. Let a thick solution of starch be made with a solution of iodide of potassium, and let strips of paper be dipped in this mixture and exposed to the free action of the air. If no ozone be present the colour of the slips is hardly affected, but when there is any appreciable quantity in the air, it liberates the iodine contained in the iodide of potassium. The free iodine now acts on the starch, and the slips assume a blue tint, whose depth and the rapidity with which the change ensues, are proportional to the amount of ozone present. Care must be taken that the slips of paper are not placed in the vicinity of cesspools, drains, or other sources of sulphuretted hydrogen, a gas which decomposes ozone.

and assumes an opaque, muco-purulent character. The breathing is short and hurried, but in most cases the sounds on auscultation are not very much modified.

The circulation is rather depressed than excited. The pulse often varies to a remarkable degree, being at one time hard and firm, and perhaps an hour or two afterwards soft and weak. This form of hard and firm pulse, however, by no means indicates the necessity for venesection; it depends on the peculiar irritation connected with this disease, not on an inflammatory state of the system.

The digestive organs are variously affected. The bowels are in some cases relaxed, in others constipated. The abdomen is tense and painful on pressure. I have already alluded to the most common appearance of the tongue.

In a few cases I have observed an almost instantaneous and universal prostration, both of bodily and mental powers, requiring the immediate and continuous use of stimulants and tonics.

I have already shown from the mortality tables that the danger from influenza is greatest in advanced life. Under the age of sixty most persons, with a little care and attention, got through the late epidemic in the course of a week or ten days, unless there was pre-existing disease of the lungs or heart. But most of the old people with whose cases I was acquainted had long and dangerous illnesses, kept their beds for a fortnight or more, and were much pulled down by the wearing character of their cough and by profuse muco-purulent expectoration. Some even at the present time (May, 1848), have continued to suffer from severe paroxysms of coughing, occurring two or three times in the twenty-four hours (especially soon after going to bed) and terminating in the expectoration of a little thick mucus; and others have not regained their former strength, and in all probability will never do so.

There is, perhaps, no disease in which greater diversities of treatment are recommended. I shall confine myself almost entirely in these remarks to the course of treatment I found most serviceable in persons of advanced life, during the late epidemic.

When called in at the commencement of the disease, I prescribed an emetic in all cases in which there was not very great prostration. It not only clears the mucous membrane of the stomach and air-tubes from the viscid secretions with which they are loaded, but it is likewise the best preparation for other remedies.

If the bowels were very torpid, a blue pill, succeeded by a mild aperient draught of rhubarb and sulphate of potash, was usually sufficient for the required object. If, on the other hand, there was diarrhœa, which in a few cases prevailed from the commencement to a very unpleasant degree, it was combated by drachm doses of castor-oil, associated with a few minims of laudanum.

The bowels being thus properly regulated, I at once had recourse to stimulating and tonic treatment. In the cases that fell under my care, I found that the best results followed the moderate use of mulled port or sherry. A wine-glassful twice a day, with a moderate allowance of good beef-tea, in no instance produced the least discomfort, or aggravated any symptom whatever; and in some cases the allowance of wine was more than trebled with advantage. I am fully aware that I may be charged with promulgating a highly dangerous mode of treatment. I willingly grant that there may be exceptional cases in which antiphlogistic measures may be demanded, but I am convinced that they are very rare, and that there is, perhaps, no other disease in which " active practice" is so fatal.

Expectorants are of little service, and sudorifics are worse than useless. The disease generally sweats the patient enough, and to spare.

I hardly know how far we can regard narcotics as indicated in this disease. While in some cases they were of undoubted service in allaying the cough, I am convinced that I have seen much harm from their indiscriminate use; as in cases in which the influenza was grafted on asthma and cardiac affections.

In the cases of extreme and sudden prostration to which I alluded, quinine and camphor were given, with wine, beef-tea, &c. from the beginning; but in the majority of instances, bark was not prescribed for the first few days. Instead of increasing the cough and tightness of the chest, it seemed often to relieve these symptoms.

Amongst the external applications found serviceable, I may mention blisters, used as counter-irritants rather than as vesicants, sinapisms, oil of turpentine, and the fomentation of the trachea and chest with very hot water applied by a sponge. I found that sponging the forehead and temples in a similar manner often afforded the greatest relief in those cases in which the headache was very distressing.

CHAPTER VIII.

DISEASES OF THE NERVOUS SYSTEM.

SECTION I.

Apoplexy and Paralysis—Mortality from these Affections—Causes giving rise to similar Head-symptoms—Hyperæmia—Anæmia—Passive Congestion of the Brain—Diminution of Nervous Energy—Apoplexy essentially a Disease of Advanced Life—Various Premonitory Symptoms—Necessity for Caution in Blood-letting—Dangers subsequent to an Apoplectic Attack—On the Treatment of the Pains occurring in Paralysed Limbs, and on the best Mode of attempting the Restoration of the suspended Nervous Functions.

Our mortality tables afford us comparatively little information regarding the deaths occurring at an advanced age from diseases of the nervous system. We learn little more from them than that during the five years extending from the beginning of 1843 to the end of 1847, 6947 deaths, at and above the age of 60, are noted as occurring in this metropolis, from this class of diseases. Of these, 2812 are ascribed to apoplexy, and 2806 to paralysis,* leaving 1329 cases to cerebral softening, diseases of the membranes, &c.

I have shown, in the table in pp. 66, 67, that diseases of the nervous system give rise to a little more than 13 per cent. of the deaths occurring at and above the age of 60.

There are various and perfectly distinct conditions which may give rise to apparently similar head-symptoms. Hyperæmia and anæmia, general debility, gout, and a poisoned condition of the blood, whether dependent on its imperfect depuration, or on the introduction of noxious agents from without, may all give rise to very similar symptoms. To these we may add certain structural changes—diseases of the heart, or of the vessels of the brain, or its membranes.

Hyperæmia is undoubtedly a common cause of those symptoms which are regarded as indicative of an approaching apoplectic attack, and when this condition is present, venesection—and copious venesection too—is undoubtedly called for. There is hardly any disease

---

* What actual information regarding the cause of death is contained in the statement that 2806 persons died from paralysis?

in which loss of blood is so well tolerated. But how are we to ascertain that hyperæmia is present? How often have we seen—more frequently some years ago than at present—hydrencephaloid disease in children mistaken for hydrocephalus! And similar mistakes too often occur in adult and advanced life. Anæmia is mistaken for hyperæmia, irritation for inflammation. Headache, vertigo, singing in the ears, and throbbing of the arteries, may arise from either of the opposite states—from an excess or a deficiency of blood. If hyperæmia is the cause of the mischief, the patient usually presents the appearance of rude health. The make of such patients is usually stout, and they are generally bull-necked. The face is flushed. There is headache, a tendency to doze, and vertigo, which becomes especially marked in stooping or in looking upwards to the ceiling of the room or the sky. Nausea is a common symptom. This form is of most frequent occurrence towards the close of middle life.

In the cases arising from anæmia we usually observe the face pale, the heart's action quick and tumultuous, and a tendency to faintness. The vertigo is most felt on suddenly assuming the upright position. There is a feeling of headache and dizziness—the patient often complaining that he feels as if an iron band were contracting his forehead. It unfortunately happens that depletion gives temporary relief, although it causes a subsequent aggravation of the symptoms. Hence it is often difficult to persuade the patient of the impropriety of bloodletting and cupping. The proper treatment—the administration of iron, quinine, &c.—is slow, although certain, in its effects.

Aged persons are liable to a peculiar form of head-affection, depending, for the most part, on passive congestion, arising from want of tone in the vascular system. Gravitation, which exerts a manifest influence on the circulation at all periods of life, and whose effects are counteracted by many beautiful provisions of nature—valves, tortuosities, &c.—remains unaffected, whilst the forces opposed to it are gradually weakened. Hence, if aged persons remain for any length of time with the head in the same position, the blood accumulates in undue quantity in the most dependent parts of the brain, and gives rise to drowsiness, sometimes approaching to coma, to partial paralysis, and to other alarming symptoms. This affection may be regarded as analogous, in its nature and treatment, to the peculiar form of pulmonary affection noticed in page 70. The brain in this, as the lung in that instance, suffers from the successful struggle of **physical** over vital forces; and it is much to be feared that too often the physician, with his depleting weapons, unconsciously sides with the enemy.

The only available practice in these cases is to vary the position of the patient with the view to guard against mechanical stases at particular parts of the brain, and unless there are obvious contra-indications to administer tonics and mild stimulants. I have found the compound infusion of horse-radish a good stimulant in these cases. The head-symptoms in fever are, I suspect, often partly dependent on this cause. We should look out for, and guard against them in all long-continued illnesses, especially when there is a want of tone in the vascular system.

There is a state of the brain, more common in advanced than in mature life, characterized by diminution or alteration of the nervous energy. The head-symptoms occurring in continued fevers, in delirium tremens, and in cases of starvation are dependent on a condition of this sort. In a less marked degree, but similar in kind, are the symptoms produced by long-continued anxiety and distress of mind, and by over-exertion of the intellectual faculties. In these cases there is a tendency to various forms of paralytic and spasmodic affections. The treatment must be the same as in the cases of anæmia already described. Venesection would most probably induce incurable paralysis.

Further remarks bearing on similar symptoms, and the mode of treatment to be adopted, will be found under the heads of Diseases of the Liver, Diseases of the Kidney, Diseases of the Skin, and Gout.

Any of the above causes, different as they essentially are, may predispose to an attack of apoplexy or paralysis.

It would be altogether foreign to the object of this volume, to enter into the general consideration of apoplexy, or of paralysis. Apoplexy is so essentially a disease of advanced life,* that the treatment recommended in all our standard works applies to it as it occurs in old age. The same remark applies, in a great measure, to paralysis; although there are certain local forms of this affection to which I shall have occasion, in various places, to refer.

Having shown that some of the most striking premonitory symptoms may arise from very different causes I shall now revert to certain additional symptoms, which may enable us to detect, and possibly avert, a threatened apoplectic attack. I have already noticed a flushed state of the countenance, a tendency to sleep, vertigo, nausea, and

* The following valuable table, from Dr. Burrow's work, "On Disorders of

headache. To these we may add wakefulness (which, however, is much rarer than the opposite state), a general incapacity for exertion, and an indescribable sensation of weight about the limbs; torpor, and numbness, or else a sensation of formication, or itching in the extremities: slight paralytic affections, as drooping of an eyelid, or distortion of the features; disordered function of the organs of the senses, as for instance, double vision, difficulty in writing in a straight line, or in reading, muscæ volitantes, or coruscations, noises in the ears, or dulness of hearing, sometimes amounting to deafness; sometimes patients assert that every thing they touch feels like velvet or felt; the substitution of one word for another, difficulty in enunciating certain words, a sudden loss of memory, an indescribable and unaccountable feeling of terror or impending danger, &c., &c.* All or any of these symptoms should put both the physician and the patient on their guard. The treatment of these symptoms, is sketched out in the preceding pages.

I have no remarks to offer on the description of the attack, and little to say regarding the treatment of it. In advanced life we must be especially careful in ascertaining the causes giving rise to the attack, before we proceed to take blood. If the heart's action be the Cerebral Circulation," affords sufficient evidence of the correctness of this statement.

Age.	Number of cases.	Population of this age.	Proportion of Cases in 1000 Persons.
20 to 30	16	3000	5·3
30 to 40	30	2500	12·0
40 to 50	40	1800	22·2
50 to 60	41	1300	31·5
60 to 70	54	1000	54·0
70 to 80	30	500	60·0
80 and upwards	4	200	
	215	10300	

The population is here assumed to be 20,000, of which about one-half will not have attained the age of twenty years.

The changes that the arterial system undergoes in advanced life (see page 35), greatly favour several forms of cerebral disease.

* Amongst other premonitory symptoms, is one to which my attention was first directed by the perusal of Dr. Graves's *Clinical Medicine,* and which, in some instances, is very well marked. I refer to what he terms *cerebral respiration.* The breathing is permanently irregular, and interrupted by frequent sighing—going on for a minute or two at one rate, then for a quarter of a minute or so at another rate. When this occurs without any disease of the chest, we have good grounds for suspecting the existence of cerebral derangement of some kind.

strong,* the head hot, and the face flushed or livid, blood may be taken from the nape of the neck, or between the shoulders, the amount being determined by the effect produced on the vascular system. In the absence of these symptoms, and when the attack is characterized by a deficiency of vital power, blood-letting, in any form, would only increase the danger. Moreover we not unfrequently meet with cases in which, although blood-letting is ultimately called for, it must be postponed till the vital powers begin to rally, and reaction ensues.

It is unnecessary to enter into the consideration of the use of purgatives and other medicines in these cases; neither does the restorative treatment required, where the attack depends on the depressed vital energy, demand special notice.

The accidents most to be dreaded, after the immediate danger is past, are fresh extravasation from excitement of the cerebral circulation, and inflammation of the brain or its membranes. These must be guarded against by a careful regulation of the diet and habits of the patient. Any excess of corporeal or mental exertion is in the highest degree dangerous, for a considerable period after an attack.

There are only two other points to which I shall advert in this section; these are, first, in reference to the treatment of the pains so often experienced in paralysed limbs, and secondly, in reference to the means of restoring the suspended functions of the nerves in these parts.

The injured state of the brain renders most of the remedies used to allay pain, in the highest degree dangerous. These pains are often very distressing, and are compared by the patients to an exaggeration of the ordinary sensation of "pins and needles." I have recently tried chloroform externally in two cases, with a more persistent effect than I recollect to have experienced from any other local application.

When we have reason to believe that the congestion or effusion is removed, a more or less paralysed state of some part of the body remains. I notice the treatment to be adopted here, because I believe it often to be injudiciously active. Regular friction with the hands and with horse-hair gloves, should have a fair trial before other means are resorted to. This should be followed by the use of mildly stimulating liniments. If these means prove unsuccessful, I then have recourse to electro-magnetism. A weak current should be used, and

* Dr. Burrows has, with much judgment, called the attention of the profession to the indications afforded by the heart, for or against free venesection. *On Disorders of the Cerebral Circulation, &c.*, pp. 140–143.

if it is found to excite much pain in the paralysed limb, there is strong probability that it is doing more harm than good. Judiciously applied, it is a most valuable remedy, and often succeeds when all other means have failed. I have scarcely ever seen any good effects from strychnine in these cases occurring in aged persons. As in the case of the electro-magnetic current, when its administration gives pain, it should be at once discontinued.

SECTION II.

MENINGEAL APOPLEXY.

THE observations in the preceding section refer to the cases in which the congestion or effusion occurs in the parenchymatous tissue of the brain. Meningeal apoplexy,* consisting, pathologically, in a sanguineous effusion into the cavity of the arachnoid, the sub-arachnoid cellular tissue, or the ventricles, now claims our attention. It is worthy of remark, that the diseases of serous membranes occupy a prominent place in the pathology of aged persons. Their predisposition to hemorrhage, and to the low inflammation already alluded to (see page 56), is most probably, in part at least, induced by the diminished action of the skin, which thus gives rise to an augmented exhalation from the serous surfaces, in just the same way as it increases the secretion of the pulmonary mucous membrane.

Of the two classes of diseases, hemorrhages are the least common, but they are far from being rare. They may occur not only in the arachnoid, the sub-arachnoid space, and the cerebral ventricles, the parts we are now considering, but also in the pleura, the pericardium and the peritoneum.

It appears, from a consideration of the recorded cases of meningeal apoplexy in aged persons, that premonitory symptoms, such as headache, drowsiness, numbness, vertigo, &c., may or not occur. (Premonitory symptoms were present in eighteen of the forty-one cases

---

* As comparatively little attention has been bestowed on this subject in England, I may refer my readers to the following monographs: Baillarger *Du siège de quelques hémorrhagies des Meninges*. Thèse de 1837. Paris: E. Boudet in the *Journ. des Conn. méd-chir*. Nov. 1838 and Feb. 1839; and Prus, in vol. xi. of the *Mémoires de l'Acad. royale de Médicine*. I should not omit to notice an excellent memoir on the morbid anatomy of this disease by Mr. Prescot Hewett.

recorded by Boudet.) The attack itself, whether there have been premonitory symptoms or not, often comes on so rapidly and severely, as to merit the expressive term of the French writers, *apoplexie foudroyante.*

Prus, in an able memoir on this affection, points out certain important differences between sub-arachnoid and intra-arachnoid hemorrhages.

In sub-arachnoid hemorrhage, even when very considerable, no paralysis either of motion or sensation is induced, when the blood is poured forth by exhalation,* or from the rupture of a vein. When the hemorrhage occurs from the rupture of an artery, paralysis sometimes occurs. The greater impulse with which blood escapes from an artery than from a vein, or from the capillaries, sufficiently explains this difference.† In intra-arachnoid hemorrhage paralysis of motion, although by no means a constant symptom, is comparatively frequent. Prus observed it six times in eight cases, but Boudet and others have found it much more seldom. Paralysis of sensation is more rare.

In sub-arachnoid hemorrhage there is *never* a sudden loss of consciousness, whereas in intra-arachnoid hemorrhage this often occurs.

In the former there are somnolence and coma, without headache, fever, dryness of the tongue, or delirium, at least in the great majority of cases; in the latter there are somnolence and coma, usually accompanied with headache, fever, dryness of the tongue, and delirium.

In the former we have neither convulsions, contraction of the limbs, nor rigidity; in the latter we have at least one of these symptoms.

These are the principal symptomatic differences between these two forms of meningeal apoplexy.

The difficulty of establishing an accurate diagnosis between these forms of apoplexy, common apoplexy, softening of the brain, and tubercular meningitis,‡ is very great. In diagnosing between meningeal and ordinary apoplexy we must be influenced by the following

---

* I use the word *exhalation* simply as a matter of convenience, in reference to those cases of hemorrhage in which no injured vessel can be detected. See Vogel's *Pathological Anatomy,* vol. i. pp. 90–91.

† On this point I may refer to the ingenious experiments of Serres, in the *Annuaire des Hôpitaux civils,* 1819. The experiments were accurately made, although the conclusions he drew from them were not altogether correct.

‡ This disease is not at all confined to childhood. It is by no means rare up to the fortieth year, and there is no reason why it should not occur at an advanced period of life, in the same manner as pulmonary tubercles are then occasionally developed.

considerations :—The two leading symptoms of the latter—the sudden loss of consciousness and paralysis—are far from constant in meningeal apoplexy. If paralysis of motion occurs, it is not so complete as in cerebral hemorrhage, and it is very seldom, and then only transiently, accompanied by paralysis of sensation. The deviation of the mouth to one side, which is of such common occurrence in ordinary apoplexy, is very rare in these cases. Both forms of meningeal apoplexy frequently assume an intermittent character, in which also they differ from ordinary apoplexy.

It is sometimes impossible to distinguish meningeal apoplexy from softening of the brain.

From the evidence afforded by the cases recorded by Prus, it appears that the duration of sub-arachnoid hemorrhage does not exceed eight days; that of intra-arachnoid hemorrhage may extend to a month, and even longer; and, indeed, this affection is occasionally susceptible of cure. Death may, however, supervene directly upon the attack.

The prognosis is obviously in the highest degree unfavourable.

With regard to the treatment, I know of no point in which it differs from that of ordinary apoplexy.

I have made no reference to the third form of meningeal apoplexy—hemorrhage into the ventricles—because we have not a sufficient number of cases on record to enable us to draw any trustworthy conclusions.

SECTION III.

CEREBRAL SOFTENING.

A Disease of Advanced Life—Division into Acute and Chronic Softening—Symptoms and Progress of Acute Softening—Symptoms and Progress of Chronic Softening—Diagnosis—Prognosis—Causes—Treatment.

ALTHOUGH cerebral softening may occur at any period of life, it undoubtedly claims to be regarded as essentially a disease of advanced age. The cases on which the following table is based are 221 in number; they are collected from the writings of Andral, Rostan, Bouillaud, Dechambre, Durand-Fardel, Fuchs, and Lallemand.

Age.	Number of Cases.	Population at this age (the whole population being 20,000).	Proportion of Cases in 1000 persons.
20 to 30	18	3000	6·0
30 to 40	14	2500	5·6
40 to 50	28	1800	15·5
50 to 60	33	1300	25·4
60 to 70	50	1000	50·0
70 to 80	64	500	128·0
80 and upwards	14	200	70·0

If the number of cases on record were larger, we should probably find that the proportional number occurring at and after the age of eighty was higher than at any earlier period of life. Some conception of its frequency may be formed from the circumstance that out of one hundred and one cases of death from diseases of the nervous system observed by Prus, twenty-three were due to cerebral softening.

In accordance with my plan of avoiding all details of pathological anatomy in this volume, I shall subdivide this disease in reference to its symptoms, rather than to the appearances found after death.

Hence we shall consider (1) *acute softening*, and (2) *chronic softening*.

Acute softening appears in more than half the recorded cases to present no premonitory symptoms, and to induce loss of consciousness, and paralysis in the same sudden manner as cerebral hemorrhage. This is termed the apoplectic form. In other cases its invasion is solely marked by a general or partial, but progressive, weakening of the intellectual faculties, and by various modifications of sensation.

When premonitory symptoms occur, they usually present themselves as intense headache, vertigo, formication, cramps, &c.

In persons of sixty and upwards the apoplectic form is the most common; there is sudden loss of consciousness, contortion of the features, and the limbs on one side are rendered more or less insensible to external impressions, and either lie immoveable and devoid of all power, or else are powerfully flexed. Persons thus attacked often die in a few days, without any return of consciousness; but in the majority of cases consciousness gradually returns, and the use of the paralysed parts is to a certain degree restored. This apparent improvement is, however, transitory and deceptive, for a progressive torpor of the intellectual faculties is soon perceived, while the paralysis extends and becomes more perfect; and the patient, if not cut off by some of the complications to which I shall presently refer, dies in a state of coma.

As the softening progresses, we sometimes (in about a quarter of the cases) have a considerable amount of frontal headache. Dulness of the intellectual faculties and loss of memory, are almost invariably to be observed; the mouth is drawn on one side, and there is often strabismus. Patients complain of cramps, pains, a sensation of cold and formication in some of the limbs, and sometimes there is partial paralysis. Contraction of one or more of the limbs is a symptom, whose importance has, I think, been overrated by Lallemand and some other authors. It certainly does not occur in half the cases of which we have authentic records.

Those who have made cerebral softening their especial study, assert that a very opposite class of symptoms is occasionally noticed; that there may be cerebral excitement, violent delirium, and convulsions.

The rapidity with which the disease runs its course is sufficiently obvious from the following table, founded on fifty-nine cases (twenty-seven of Durand-Fardel, sixteen of Rostan, and sixteen of Andral).

Death occurred 11 times during the first two days.
" 26 times before the fifth day.
" 43 times before the ninth day.
" 7 times between the ninth and the twentieth days.
" 9 times between the twentieth and thirtieth days.

Death is seldom preceded by any febrile symptoms. It occasionally happens that the disease merges into the chronic form; and sometimes, but very rarely, there is a gradual remission of the symptoms, and a restoration to perfect health.

Chronic softening presents the same class of symptoms as those we have already described. In the majority of these cases, the patient complains of a feeling of discomfort, headache, vertigo, and stupor, which may last for weeks and months; then follow more marked symptoms—difficulty in speaking, numbness, formication or pricking of the limbs, and especially of the fingers, partial loss of power and motion, shown, for instance, in one leg dragging in walking, or in the inability to grasp objects firmly.

Contraction of the limbs in these chronic cases is much more frequent than entire loss of power, whereas the reverse holds good in acute softening: it must not, however, be regarded as a constant symptom, being absent in at least one-fourth of all the recorded cases; neither must it be regarded as a certain diagnostic sign of this disease; it is met with in connexion with disease of the membranes without any affection of the cerebral substance, in cases of mere cerebral irritation, &c. Pains in the limbs and joints generally accompany these contractions; they are usually much aggravated by motion, but not increased on pressure. There is commonly a partial, but scarcely ever a perfect loss of sensation in the paralysed and flexed limbs. The face becomes partially drawn aside, and the features are devoid of expression. The memory is gradually lost, the ideas become confused, and all reasoning power disappears. It becomes difficult to speak, in part from the required words being forgotten, and in part from loss of control over the organs of speech. The mental condition of the patient is but a few shades superior to that of the idiot. The paralysis gradually extends, the power of retaining the contents of the bladder and rectum disappears, the limbs waste away, and yet the force with which they are flexed is almost incredible, and thus the patient sinks, utterly unconscious of his own pitiable condition. In some cases the flexure ceases and the limbs relax shortly before death.

Such are the ordinary symptoms of chronic softening. We occasionally however meet with cases in which extensive softening is revealed after death, but in which no perceptible symptom is appreciable during life; and again, in which some time previous to death the symptoms have much abated.

Nothing very definite can be said regarding the duration of chronic softening; I believe it may go on for years. Death takes place in various ways; it is often dependent on the supervention of a more active head-affection, and coma or convulsions close the scene; meningitis may be developed, or there may be cerebral or meningeal hemorrhage, or an abundant effusion of serum into the ventricles or the sub-arachnoid space. Many patients finally sink from pneumonia, or in consequence of bed-sores on the sacrum.

I have thus noticed, separately, the symptoms and progress of the two great forms of cerebral softening. The remaining observations have reference to both forms.

That there are often great difficulties in the diagnosis of cerebral softening is a fact beyond all question; it may be mistaken for inflammation of the brain or of its membranes, for congestion, for cerebral or meningeal apoplexy, or for morbid growths or deposits in the brain. The diagnosis must be determined by the weighing of opposite probabilities.

Although the prognosis must always be most unfavourable, especially in the chronic form, there is undoubted evidence that the disease is occasionally cured. Cases sometimes occur in which all the symptoms we have described gradually disappear, and where there is an almost perfect return of sensation, and of the power of the intellect, and of motion.

What are the causes of cerebral softening? No definite reply can be given to this question, but it is so often associated with arterial disease (atheromatous and calcareous deposits in the smaller arteries of the brain), and is I believe so dependent on it, that the primary cause of the alteration in the structure of the arteries, may also be said to be the primary cause of cerebral softening.* I look upon the disease as consisting essentially in a perverted or diminished nutrition, somewhat analogous to that which occurs in senile gangrene.

It only remains to speak of the treatment; having established our diagnosis to the best of our power (for I believe that a certain diagnosis is occasionally impossible) all we can do (or at least do without increasing the risk of the patient) is to treat symptoms. When the disease commences with symptoms of congestion, purgatives, and the frequent application of leeches to the anus constitute the safest treatment. A seton or issue in the back of the neck, has been found serviceable in a more advanced stage. In the atonic form of the disease, we may do temporary good by mildly nourishing food and tonics.

The paralysis dependent on softening is never relieved by external applications or by strychnine.

* Eisenmann (*Die Hirnerweichung*, 1842) is I think correct in regarding cerebral softening as the result of various distinct morbid conditions, rather than as a specific disease. Amongst the causes of softening of the brain, he places (1) mechanical influences, (2) miasmatic influences, namely, rheumatic, erysipelatous and typhous miasmata, or the atmospheric influences inducing these diseases, (3) chronic dyscrasiæ, (4) uræmia (5) pyæmia, (6) the abuse of spirituous drinks, (7) disturbance in the circulation, (8) scrofulous tumours, apoplectic cysts, &c., in the brain, (9) various conditions depending on advanced life, and (10) the influence of a diseased spinal cord.

SECTION IV.

MENINGITIS.

A frequent and dangerous Disease in Old Persons; — Symptoms—Progress—Causes—Diagnosis—Treatment.

ACUTE meningitis is considered by Schönlein* to be so common in old persons that he regards it as essentially a disease of declining life. It was the cause of 25 out of 101 deaths, arising from disease of the nervous system (Prus). My own experience leads me to believe that it is less common in this country, than it seems to be in Germany and France. There are some few points in which it differs from the meningitis of earlier life. It comes on with a much less marked train of symptoms, than in infancy or middle life. In the morning, an old person is perhaps observed to be dull and stupid; the intelligence is scarcely affected, but there is a slowness in combining the ideas; the tongue is dry and there is a slight fever, but the heat of the body does not seem increased, except over the region of the forehead; and there is headache. In the evening the temperature of the body is higher, and the conjunctiva is injected, and there is most commonly a slight degree of delirium, the patient generally giving incoherent replies to questions addressed to him. In other cases although patients may answer questions correctly, they behave in an irrational manner. If the disease is not successfully combated in its early stage, they fall into a state of somnolence or coma, and death generally ensues in a period varying from five days to three weeks. Such is the most common form of meningitis in old persons. As a general rule, the period of invasion, which in early and middle life is well marked, either does not occur or is so slight as to be unobserved in advanced life; and indeed the cases are by no means rare in which an examination of the body after death, shows that meningitis has existed to a very considerable extent, without exciting any disturbance of the intellectual faculties, or of the movements of the body.

In some cases, sopor is the first symptom, coming on suddenly and not associated with paralysis or any obvious indication of congestion. It is difficult to rouse the patient from this state; he complains of ver-

* *Allgemeine und specielle Pathologie und Therapie*, 3d Ed., vol. i. p. 200.

tigo, and cannot hold up his head. The bowels are constipated and the urine is very scanty. There is always a considerable degree of fever in these cases.

When the disease terminates in a cure, the sopor gradually diminishes; but the intellectual faculties usually remain torpid for some time. As a general rule the prognosis is very unfavourable.

It is often impossible to ascertain the cause of this affection. Intemperate habits, especially when associated with exposure to cold and wet, may be regarded as predisposing causes. It frequently succeeds injuries of the head, apoplexy, exposure to a powerful sun, fits of drunkenness, or a violent revulsion of feeling. Moreover it is of no uncommon occurrence in certain forms of disease, especially in pneumonia, Bright's disease, peritonitis, pleurisy, facial erysipelas, and acute articular rheumatism.

The diagnosis of this disease may generally be established with tolerable certainty, if due attention be paid to the collective symptoms.* The diseases most liable to be mistaken for it, are low typhoid fever, gout in the head, and some forms of pneumonia. It may be laid down as a general rule, that when an old person in previous apparent health, presents signs of delirium, either in his conversation or in his actions, complains of severe headache, and has a dry, brown tongue, without there being any condition of the thoracic or abdominal viscera to account for those symptoms, we should be on the watch for further indications of meningitis.

The treatment must be active, and if the heart's action be tolerably strong and regular, blood must be taken from the arm. This is one of the very few cases in which general is preferable to local bleeding in old persons. Leeches in relays may afterwards be applied to the mastoid processes. The head must be kept cool and somewhat elevated; the bowels must be kept well open, and the treatment must be in the full sense of the word antiphlogistic. The disease is a most dangerous one, and is too often beyond the reach of any treatment.

Further remarks on the gouty form of meningitis are given in Chapter XIII.

* Systematic treatises on Medicine tell us that meningitis may be confounded with (1) tubercular meningitis, (2) cerebral congestion or hemorrhage, (3) epilepsy, (4) tetanus, (5) mania, (6) acute delirium, (7) delirium tremens, (8) eruptive fevers, (9) dentition, (10) pneumonia, (11) puerperal fevers, (12) phlebitis, (13) ataxic typhoid fevers, and (14) misplaced gout.

SECTION V.

On the Mental Diseases of Advanced Life.

The present chapter could hardly be deemed complete without a brief notice of the forms of mental derangement to which persons in the declining years of life, are especially liable. MM. Esquirol and Leuret, have arrived at the conclusion, from the evidence afforded them by 12,869 cases, that the probability of insanity increases with advancing years (plus l'homme avance dans la vie plus il est exposé à la perte de la raison). There are four forms which may be characterized as specially belonging to the period of life, of which this volume treats.

1. Insanity connected with the cessation of the menstrual discharge, with the suppression of hemorrhages, or with the rapid healing of ulcers or skin diseases.

2. Insanity depending probably on a diseased condition of the cerebellum, or of the prostate in men, and of the ovaries or uterus in women, and exhibiting itself in abnormal, or excessive erotic desires. "Abnormal erotic propensities," says one of our most philosophic writers on insanity, Dr. Prichard, "have given rise to a series of phenomena in human actions, which have been considered to belong to the province of the moralist, or the enactor of penal chastisements, rather than to that of the medical philosopher. That this opinion has been founded in error we are fully convinced, and we doubt not that the time will come, when the very names of many offences against decorum, now considered punishable crimes, will be erased from the statute-book; and when persons, now liable to be sentenced to the pillory or the gallows, will be treated as lunatics."

The treatment in these cases is sufficiently obvious, when we can ascertain the cause of the irritation. It too often happens that the disease is overlooked till the patient is led on to some gross outrage on public decorum.

3. Insanity usually commencing about the age of sixty, without reference to sex, and apparently connected pathologically with the altered character of the cerebral circulation, that generally supervenes

about that period. This form has been admirably described by Dr. Seymour.*

The patient becomes morose, is exceedingly distressed and annoyed about trifles, and frequently has gloomy forebodings of the future. He suspects his old and best friends, fancies there are conspiracies against him, or has a morbid fear of dying a pauper. We must beware of suicide in these cases. I have been recently consulted regarding the case of a rich old gentleman about 70 years of age, of sanguineous temperament and strong frame, who made a large fortune by his own exertions, and for the last six or seven years has retired from business. With no definite object or resource, he has spent his leisure days in pondering over the horrors of a speedy chartist rule in England, and this predominant idea is so strangely mixed up with so strong a feeling of the extreme necessity for economy, that although he would on no account dispense with a good dinner and the most expensive wines, there is the greatest difficulty in persuading him to *pay* for the most necessary articles of life. The smallest demand for money is instantly suggestive of the workhouse, which unfortunately for the poor old gentleman's happiness is actually visible from his library window.

The treatment recommended consisted essentially in an increased amount of exercise in the open air (chiefly horse exercise); alternate cupping from the nape of the neck, and leeches to the anus at intervals of a month or six weeks; a sufficient dose of a mixture of the common black draught and compound decoction of aloes, to insure at least two motions; and an opiate at bedtime.

He has now been under this course of treatment for about two months, and I hear that his temper is much improved, that the moroseness and gloominess have altogether disappeared, and although the principal delusions are not altogether removed, that he regards the impending miseries of his country, as a due and proper retribution, ordained by a wise providence, for the passing of the Reform Bill. I entertain strong hopes of his further improvement.

4. Senile dementia or fatuity. For a clear perception of this condition I must briefly notice certain points connected with the ordinary state of the mind in old persons.

The intellectual powers usually remain unimpaired longer than the physical. We find however that the mind (*the spiritual life* of Can-

* *Thoughts on the Nature and Treatment of several severe Diseases of the Human Body*, Vol. I. p. 187, &c.

statt and other German writers) seems rather to live on the matters hoarded up in past times, than to continue to absorb fresh nutriment through the external senses ; for the organs of these senses have undergone physical alterations, and the impressions conveyed to the brain are, as it were, dimmed and blunted. Hence while his judgment and opinion on the things and times of his youth are usually correct, the old man is liable to arrive at very incorrect results regarding the things occurring around him. Whilst his remembrance of the acts of yesterday is blotted out, the recollections of his childhood and youth are strong and deep. Living almost solely in the reminiscences of the past, the present holds out no attractions for him. He feels that the years, so graphically described in sacred writ, have come, " when thou shalt say, I have no pleasure in them," when " the grasshopper shall be a burden, and desire shall fail."

Let us briefly trace the gradual decline of the mental faculties in so far as it bears on this question. I have already mentioned the order in which memory is first affected. In the words of Dr. Holland,* (1) the faculty of receiving and associating fresh impressions for the most part declines earlier than the power of combining and using those formerly received ; and (2) the faculty of directing and fixing combinations or successions of ideas, is one of those earliest impaired. In some cases, a word, or even part of a word, of double application, will suddenly and without the consciousness of change, carry off the mind to a new and wholly foreign subject ; and in others, in which the memory is remarkably tenacious as to persons and detailed events of past life, there is a singular incapacity of associating them together by any reasonable link ; and the slightest relations of time or place suffice to carry the mind wholly astray from its subject. In reference to the decay of memory, the power of recollecting words and names is lost earlier and more readily than that of events ; the ideas are often sufficiently distinct while the words required for their expression are either not forthcoming, or others in no way applicable are substituted.† Defining senile dementia as a decay of the mental

---

* *Medical Notes and Reflections*, 2d Ed. p. 288, Note.

† "The first case of this kind, which occurred to me in practice, was that of an attorney, much respected for his integrity and talents, but who had many sad failings to which our physical nature too often subjects us. Although nearly in his 70th year, and married to an amiable lady, much younger than himself, he kept a mistress whom he was in the habit of visiting every evening. The arms of Venus are not wielded with impunity at the age of 70. He was suddenly

faculties, it is obvious that the preceding remarks furnish us with an almost perfect history of the disease in question. It begins with dulness of perception or apprehension. The mind seems unable fully to recognise the ideas, somewhat dimly presented to it, through the organs of the senses. " Perception indeed takes place, but the impression is momentarily evanescent. The individual sees and hears; he replies to questions, but his attention is so little excited that he speedily forgets what he has said, and repeats the same remarks or inquries after a few minutes. At the same time ideas long ago impressed upon the mind, remain nearly in their original freshness, and are capable of being called up whenever the attention is directed towards them.

"Sensations produced by present objects are so slight and the notions connected with them so confused and indistinct, that the individual affected scarcely knows where he is; yet he recognises without difficulty persons with whom he has long been acquainted, and if questioned regarding his former life, and the transactions and pursuits of his youth or manhood, he will often give pertinent and sensible replies. The disorder of his mind consists not in defective memory of the past, but in the incapacity for attention and for receiving the influence of present external agencies, which in a different state of the cerebral organization, would have produced a stronger effect upon the sensorium."*

Senile dementia is not the universal lot of old persons, although, as I have already remarked, there is a general tendency towards that state.

seized with a great prostration of strength, giddiness, forgetfulness, insensibility to all concerns of life, and every symptom of approaching fatuity. His forgetfulness was of the kind alluded to. When he wished to ask for any thing, he constantly made use of some inappropriate term. Instead of asking for a piece of bread, he would probably ask for his boots; but if these were brought, he knew they did not correspond with the idea he had of the thing he wished to have, and was therefore angry; yet he would still demand some of his boots or shoes, meaning bread. If he wanted a tumbler to drink out of, it was a thousand to one, he did not call for a certain chamber utensil; and if it was the said utensil he wanted, he would call it a tumbler, or a dish. He evidently was conscious that he pronounced the wrong words, for when the proper expressions were spoken by another person, and he was asked if it was not such a thing he wanted, he always seemed aware of his mistake, and corrected himself, by adopting the appropriate expression. This gentleman was cured of his complaint by large doses of valerian, and other proper medicines."—Crichton's *Inquiry into the Nature and Origin of Mental Derangement*, vol. i. p. 371.

* Prichard's *Treatise on Insanity*, pp. 89, 90.

This altered condition of the mental faculties may be accelerated by various causes, amongst which may be especially mentioned:

(1) Prolonged mental exertion.
(2) The too free use of wine or spirits.
(3) Venereal excesses. (See note to page 119.)

It often follows slight attacks of apoplexy and paralysis; its progress is then very rapid.

When the affection is once firmly established, I believe all treatment to be unavailing or nearly so. Mild tonic treatment with due attention to hygienic precautions is all that can be suggested.

Of the senile insanity described by Dr. Burrows,* I have no personal experience. It appears to differ in several points from the third form I have described.

SECTION VI.

PAINFUL AFFECTIONS OF THE NERVES.

Neuralgia generally—Its Comparative Frequency at different Periods of Life—Facial Neuralgia, or Tic Douloureux—Cervico-brachial Neuralgia—Dorso-intercostal Neuralgia—Sciatica—Treatment.

ALTHOUGH painful affections of the nerves cannot be regarded as included amongst those diseases which specially pertain to old age, they are very common in the earlier periods of declining life. The following table is in part taken from Valleix' work on Neuralgia, and partly calculated in the same manner as the tables in pages 106 and 111:—

Age.	Number of Cases.	Population at this Age.	Proportion of Cases in 1000 Persons.
10 to 20	22	3700	6·0
20 to 30	68	3000	22·7
30 to 40	67	2500	26·8
40 to 50	64	1800	35·5
50 to 60	47	1300	36·2
60 to 70	21	1000	21·0
70 to 80	5	500	10·0
	294	13800	

* *Commentaries on the Causes, Forms, Symptoms, and Treatment of Insanity*, p. 409.

From this table it appears that neuralgia is *relatively* most common between the ages of 50 and 60; its comparative rarity after that age is dependent on the peculiar condition of the nervous system to which I have alluded in page 58. It may however occur at any age, however advanced.

I shall now briefly notice some of the special seats of neuralgia.

1. *Neuralgia of the fifth pair; Facial neuralgia or Tic-douloureux*, is by no means a rare affection in persons of a declining or advanced age.* In the 119 cases collected by Chaponniere,† seventeen occurred between the ages of 50 and 60, eleven between 60 and 70, and four between 70 and 80.

Thouret‡ relates the case of a lady aged 85 years, who had suffered from facial neuralgia for upwards of thirty years, and that of another lady, attacked with it at the age of 78. Dr. Hunt refers to the case of a lady between 80 and 90 years of age; Dr. Haughton to that of a lady aged 70; Swan to that of a lady of 80; and many others might be adduced.

Although it is not my intention to enter into the diagnosis of the various forms of neuralgia, seeing that generally there is no particular difficulty on this score, peculiar to advanced life, I may take this opportunity of recommending the practitioner always to examine the mouth of the patient. When some of the teeth have fallen out, those that remain often irritate the opposite gum, and give rise to small but very painful ulcers, which in some instances have led to a very incorrect diagnosis and mode of treatment.

2. *Cervico-brachial neuralgia.*—The reader will find several well-marked cases of this affection, occurring between the ages of 62 and 70, in Valleix' *Traité des Neuralgies*, p. 289.

If the eight cases given by that author, can be deemed to afford any evidence regarding the period of life at which this affection is most common, they favour the idea of its being a disease of advanced rather than of mature age; for putting aside two cases of the respective ages of 23 and 38 years, the ages of the other patients were 50, 58, 60, 70, and 80.

---

* Attention has been drawn by Mr. Swan to the fact that when old persons complain suddenly of pain in the nerves of the face, the affection may depend on augmented vascularity of the brain, at the points from whence the nerves arise. May we not sometimes bring to a climax the existing apoplectic tendency by the means (iron, &c.) we are using against the neuralgia?

† *Essai sur le siège et les causes des Neuralgies de la Face*, 1832.

‡ *Histoire de la Societé Royale de Médicine*, Vol. II.

3. *Dorso-intercostal neuralgia.*—This may attack either one or both sides of the chest, and may extend over a single intercostal space or many; five or six are usually affected, and the fifth, sixth, seventh, eighth, and ninth, are those most commonly involved. This form of neuralgia is comparatively rare in advanced life, for of 62 cases collected by Bassereau and Valleix, there were only four between 50 and 60, and four above the age of 60. These neuralgic pains sometimes alternate with herpetic eruptions.

4. *Femoro-popliteal neuralgia or sciatica*, is perhaps of all others the form of neuralgia we are most frequently called upon to treat in persons of advanced life. Statistical data show that it is actually most frequent between the ages of 40 and 50, but relatively so (taking into consideration the different proportion of persons at different ages), between 50 and 60; and it is by no means rare afterwards.

These are the most common forms of neuralgia that we are called upon to treat in old people.

The treatment is much the same as in adult life. In neuralgia of the fifth pair, or tic-douloureux, we may sometimes find that a carious tooth is the cause of the whole mischief. The remedy in that case is a simple one. I have seen relief in some instances from the prolonged employment of a current from the galvano-magnetic machine, and I have repeatedly alleviated the intense pain by the local application of chloroform and of tincture of aconite. We occasionally however find cases in which the skin of old persons seems to act as case-armour against all external agents. There undoubtedly are cases in which the excision of the nerve has been the only means of relief.

Before adopting any specific internal treatment it is imperatively necessary to unload the abdominal viscera and clear the intestinal tube. One or two emetics and a couple of active cathartics (apportioned of course to the age and strength of the patient), often prepare the system for the successful administration of remedies, which, without this preparatory course, would only aggravate the evil. From whatever cause the tic arises,—whether from hyperæmia, or anæmia; irritation of a part at a distance from, but connected with the seat of pain; malaria, cold, and damp; or from almost any other cause,— (and we have not thought it necessary to enter into this part of the subject), this preliminary measure should never be neglected.

Amongst the most approved medicines we may mention the *pilules de Meglin*, consisting of a grain each, of extract of henbane, powdered valerian root, and oxide of zinc, valerian in other forms, valerianate of zinc, oil of turpentine, and the preparations of iron and arsenic.

When any form of neuralgia is connected with a gouty tendency, colchicum, either alone or combined with a sedative, should be prescribed. When the disease puts on an intermittent character, quinine and arsenic are the medicines to be relied on.

I have never seen any harm from the administration of cannabis indica to deaden the sensation of pain; and in many respects I prefer it to opium.

For cervico-brachial or cervico-occipital neuralgia, the line of treatment is much the same as that we have already described. A continuous series of blisters, hardly kept on sufficiently long to vesicate, is often of great service in these cases, but nothing affords such perfect and often instantaneous relief as the *thermic treatment* explained in the Appendix to this volume.

In dorso-intercostal neuralgia, we generally speaking find that internal remedies are of considerably less service, than in the forms we have described. We must trust here to the thermic treatment, or to a series of blisters applied in the way I have described.

Much has been written on the treatment of sciatica. It is a disease often very difficult to overcome, and one that requires much patience, both on the part of the sufferer and the physician. If I were compelled to adhere to a single remedy, it would unquestionably be to the thermic treatment, and, next to that, to the frequent application of blisters (as already described) to the most painful spots. In order, however, to give the latter remedy a fair chance, the patient should be confined to his bed or sofa, and should be kept comfortably warm. The bowels should be duly regulated, for which purpose (if the preliminary treatment mentioned in page 123 has been adopted), confection of senna with a little sulphur is sufficient; and a mild, nutritious, but not stimulating diet should be allowed.

I have now tried the thermic treatment with almost uniform success, in a large number of cases, in patients of all ages, and suffering under various painful local affections, and I am persuaded that the practitioner, who will first satisfy himself that the pain is unconnected with acute inflammation, or with any structural lesion, will not be disappointed in his trial of this remedy. The mode of applying it is fully explained in the Appendix. The instrument, a small flat iron button, is gently warmed in the flame of a spirit-lamp, and scarcely ever raises a blister; the operation is over in a few seconds, and as far as my experience yet goes, it is the least troublesome, the least painful, and the most effectual method of counter-irritation.

Another great advantage of this mode of treatment lies in the circumstance, that it is not necessarily associated with confinement to the sofa, or even to the house. For cases of its successful application to sciatica I must refer to the Appendix. I should add, that no internal treatment, with the exception of an emetic and warm purgative, was adopted.

Electricity has proved serviceable in my hands, in cases where the disease was of long standing, and the patients were unable to enjoy perfect quiet.

I am not in a position to offer an opinion on the therapeutic value of acupuncture. I have seen it occasionally tried successfully, as a remedy for sciatica and lumbago, but should not feel inclined to recommend it in old persons, till many other means have been found useless.

As an internal remedy I place more reliance on oil of turpentine, than on any other medicine, except in the cases connected with gout, when sciatica *must be treated as gout*,* or where there is a marked intermittence, when quinine, or, that failing, arsenic must be resorted to.

There is a singular class of neuralgic pains which are apparently connected with diseases of the urinary organs. They are noticed in Chapter XI.

CHAPTER IX.

DISEASES OF THE DIGESTIVE TUBE AND ITS APPENDAGES.

SECTION I.

Relative Frequency of this Class of Diseases—Loss of Appetite—Flatulence—Constipation—Aphthous Eruptions—Dysphagia—Pyrosis—Indigestion—Cholera—Senile Gastritis—Cancer of the Stomach.

THE diseases of the digestive system do not stand nearly so prominently forward in the Mortality Tables as the diseases of the respiratory and nervous systems. It is shown in pp. 66, 67, that of 1000

* In cases where colchicum alone has failed, colchicum and quinine have rapidly succeeded in effecting a cure.

deaths at and above the age of 60, about 59 are dependent on this class of diseases, and if to these we add the deaths from diarrhœa, which is commonly a disease of the blood, although its effects are principally manifested in the altered state of the intestinal secretions, we only raise the mortality from diseases of the digestive system to 79·5 in 1000 deaths at or above 60.

Prus in the monograph to which I have already alluded, found on examining the bodies of 390 aged persons, that death resulted in 49 cases from diseases of the digestive canal and its peritoneal coat, and in 8 from disease of the liver and gall-bladder. A slight calculation will show that these numbers yield a result nearly twice as high as that of our London tables, or about 146 in 1000. In the cases examined by Prus, death arose 27 times from enteritis, 10 times from cancer of the stomach, 4 times from gastro-enteritis, 3 times from dysentery, and 3 times from hepatitis, leaving 10 miscellaneous cases.

My remarks on this class of disorders are necessarily of a very discursive character, and in many cases I have treated of symptoms rather than actual diseases.

A peculiar *loss of appetite*, altogether distinct from the anorexia resulting from gastric disturbance is sometimes observed in advanced life. It is dependent on weakness and want of tone in the digestive organs, and must be treated by aromatics and bitter tonics. Half a glass of Madeira, shortly before dinner, is often of service in these cases.

Flatulence is very common at this period, and is often so severe as to give rise to sleeplessness, asthmatic paroxysms, palpitations, and vertigo. The mucous membrane of the stomach and intestines sometimes secretes a large quantity of gas, which gives rise to very annoying symptoms. The diet must be carefully regulated by the physician in these cases. Our treatment must be directed against the atonic condition of the digestive organs, and the congested state of the portal circulation. Temporary relief is usually afforded by the administration of two drops of cajeput oil on a lump of sugar, or of a pill containing a grain of cayenne pepper. The bowels should at the same time be regulated by confection of senna to which may be added sulphur, bitartrate of potash, or confection of black pepper, according to circumstances; and the general tone of the system be kept up by vegetable, or the milder metallic tonics, cold water injections, &c.

The distention of the stomach from flatulence is often attended with very alarming symptoms, as convulsions or apoplexy. In these cases mustard poultices must be applied to the pit of the stomach, and we must administer the compound infusion of horse-radish, and repeated draughts of very hot water.

We have already noticed the importance of attending to the due regulation of the bowels (see page 51); we now proceed to consider more fully the subject of constipation in persons of advanced life.

Constipation may occur in old persons from two distinct causes, from a want of tone in the muscular fibres, or from a deficient secretion of mucus.

The modes of treatment most to be relied on, in severe cases of the first form of constipation, are the passage of a mild galvano-magnetic current from the mouth to the anus, and the combination of small doses of extract of nux vomica or strychnine with the ordinary purgatives. We must however be careful to see that there is no great accumulation of fæces in the lower bowels, as in that case we can expect little service from the treatment I have recommended. Oleaginous purgatives must then be given both by the mouth and by the rectum, and their use must be continued for some time. Numerous cases occur in which hardened fæces accumulate in the lower part of the intestinal canal, and can only be removed after being broken down by a scoop, or other appropriate instrument.

When constipation is dependent on an insufficient secretion of mucus, it may frequently be obviated by simple dietetic means. In cases where these have failed, I have usually found that small doses of croton oil, repeated for a few days in combination with a mild aperient pill, stimulate the follicles and give rise to an augmentation of the mucous secretion.

In all cases we must attempt to regulate the bowels by the mildest means. If they remain costive, after two or three doses of purgative medicine, we must be very careful how we carry out the ordinary plan of trying more powerful remedies. Emollient enemata furnish us with the safest line of treatment in these cases.

I have been frequently consulted by patients of sixty years and upwards, respecting *aphthous eruptions of the mouth*. They occur for the most part on the interior of the cheeks, and on the tongue, and possibly extend, although unseen, over a considerable extent of the mucous membrane. I have chiefly observed them in persons in whom there is an excessive development of acidity, and in those in whom the blood appears to be impoverished.

There is always more or less gastric disturbance in these cases, which must be combated before the local symptoms give way. The most serviceable local application is nitrate of silver.

Dysphagia or pain and difficulty in the act of deglutition not unfrequently induces old people to seek medical assistance. It may be dependent on two very separate and distinct causes, namely, on an atonic or paralytic condition of the œsophagus, or on the occurrence of malignant disease in or near that organ.

The atonic form of dysphagia seems dependent on a loss of power in the muscular fibres of the œsophagus, and occasionally in the muscles of the pharynx.

The most striking symptoms are difficulty in swallowing, but no pain or feeling of constriction. The respiration is unaffected, and no tumour pressing on the canal can be perceived on examination. Solids are swallowed with more ease than fluids; and I am acquainted with cases in which highly seasoned dishes were the only food that could be swallowed with any degree of ease. Might not this have arisen from the local stimulus of the condiments on the paralysed organs?—and hence a clue to the treatment.

This form of dysphagia occasionally assumes a periodic character. But whether continued or intermittent, it must be carefully watched, as it is not unfrequently the precursor of more extended paralysis or apoplexy.

As a general rule stimulating applications are the most serviceable. The thermic treatment or blisters may be applied to the neck and down the vertebral column; stimulating gargles may be prescribed, and the patient may be directed to chew horse-radish or ginger, and to swallow his saliva. Amongst other means the endermic application of strychnine, douches over the cervical vertebræ, and electricity have also found their advocates.

The other form of dysphagia is dependent on contraction of the œsophagus, caused by the deposition of cancerous matter in the soft structures of that organ, or by tumours in the immediate vicinity.

Severe pain is usually felt at the spot where the contraction exists.

As soon as the food reaches the stricture, the most agonising pain is often excited. The patient experiences the sensation of impending suffocation, and the food itself is ejected, covered with a tough mucopurulent fluid. In this form of dysphagia fluids are more easily swallowed than solids. Death by starvation or slow fever, usually terminates the scene.

Our treatment in these cases can only be palliative.

Pyrosis or *water-brash* is not an uncommon affection in advanced life, especially in persons who have been addicted to spirit-drinking. It is often a premonitory symptom of cancer of the stomach or of dilatation of that organ; but is sometimes dependent merely on an atonic condition of that viscus; and I have known it connected with disease of the pancreas.

It must be regarded in the light of a symptom rather than as a disease, and our treatment must be directed to the primary seat of the morbid action. When dependent on irritation of the gastric mucous membrane, I have found most service from creosote, and from combinations of astringents and narcotics, such as the compound kino powder.

The symptoms we have just noticed are all of them more or less connected with *indigestion* generally. I have already alluded (in page 35) to some of the reasons why indigestion is common in advanced life, and I shall now offer a few remarks on *senile dyspepsia* generally, and on its most appropriate treatment. It is an affection presenting itself in the most varied forms; it may be acute or chronic; and accompanied by, or free from fever. In the winter it is usually associated with chronic bronchitis and sometimes with head-affections; in the summer it is comparatively uncomplicated.

The varieties of dyspepsia most common in advanced life are the *embarras gastrique* of the French writers, which may be regarded as *acute atonic dyspepsia*, and the form which has been described by Dr. T. J. Todd as *follicular gastric dyspepsia*.

The following is a brief summary of the leading symptoms of *acute atonic dyspepsia*. The patients complain of a perfect loss of appetite, and experience a feeling of disgust towards food, especially animal, or any oily food. There is usually much thirst, and a desire is manifested for acid drinks. There is a bad taste, bitter or sour, in the mouth, which seems to communicate itself to every thing they swallow. There are nausea and vomiting. There is a peculiarly fetid and characteristic odour in the breath. The tongue is moist, and thickly covered with a yellow coating, which is partially extended in a thin layer over the teeth and gums. A tickling sensation in the back of the throat, giving rise to a continual desire to expectorate, is frequently noticed. There is a feeling of weight, amounting on pressure to actual pain in the epigastric region and extending towards the sternum. In some cases there is constipation, in others diarrhœa; and generally more or less colic. The urine is scanty, of a deep red colour, and often contains bile-pigment. The face presents a dull yellowish tint. There is a feeling of weight in the head, and the patient usually complains of frontal headache. He is extremely sensible of cold, and complains of slight chills and rigors. He is knocked up, feels sore, just as if he had been bruised all over, and is utterly incapable of any exertion, either intellectual or corporeal. He either cannot sleep, or else his sleep is unrefreshing and disturbed by horrid dreams. The pulse is rarely affected. The skin is dry, but not hot, and sometimes presents herpetic or furuncular eruptions.

This affection is often sporadic, and is most common during the latter part of the summer and the beginning of autumn.

The treatment is very simple. It consists in the administration of an emetic of ipecacuanha, or of an emeto-cathartic of a grain and a half of tartar emetic combined with a purgative salt. One emetic is generally sufficient. The patient must be kept on low and very mild diet for the first day or two. If he complains of thirst and has a dry skin, we may order soda water and a warm bath. We must then allow him some cooling aromatic water, as for instance spearmint water, and very gradually proceed to the milder vegetable tonics and more nourishing food. The bowels must be at first regulated by injections, as we should avoid any chance of irritating the mucous membrane of the stomach: and for some time subsequently by stomachic aperients, as rhubarb and magnesia or soda in some aromatic water; or if there are indications of much disturbance in the large intestine the compound decoction of aloes is preferable.

Follicular gastric dyspepsia differs in many respects from the preceding form. It is distinguished by an aching pain or sensation of gnawing and weight, felt chiefly in the morning, or at other times when the stomach is empty, by loss of appetite, but not the same disgust for food that we mentioned in the previous page, by nausea, and sometimes by the vomiting of a transparent, viscid, tasteless fluid, mixed with the fragments of undigested food. The pulse is seldom accelerated, and is usually soft; the tongue is foul, and often presents a sodden appearance, but has not the thick yellow coating described in the other form; neither is the skin so dry; indeed it is often freely covered with perspiration. Flatulence, the frequent eructation of a mawkish or faintly acid liquid, a superabundance of fluid in the mouth, either from the salivary glands or the mucous follicles, and oppression of the stomach, usually accompany this disorder. There is sometimes a frequent craving for food, and there is usually some thirst; but the act of eating is succeeded by pain or uneasiness, which gradually subsides as the process of digestion approaches its conclusion. Before, however, the proper time for again taking food has arrived, the stomach becomes irritated by its own secretion, which gives rise to the symptoms of a foreign indigestible substance in that organ; such as to feelings of sinking, of weight, of gnawing, and often of nausea and faintness, which are again for a time relieved by the taking of food. The bowels are generally confined, and large quantities of mucus are sometimes mixed with the scanty motions. The urine is high coloured, but not sedimentary so often as might be expected.

Amongst the sympathetic affections which are associated with, and characterize this form of dyspepsia, we almost always observe a troublesome cough which is much increased by taking food, and considerable dyspnœa, which is partly dependent on the sympathetic condition of the bronchial mucous membrane, and partly on the flatulent distention of the stomach. Headache is comparatively rare.

The disease consists in a disordered state of the mucous follicles, which may however depend upon very opposite conditions of the mucous membrane—on an anæmic or congested state. In either case there is an abnormal secretion of mucus; and that the accumulation of this substance is the proximate cause of much of the painful sensations in this form of dyspepsia, seems obvious from the relief afforded by its ejection.

The treatment consists essentially in a due regulation of the diet in reference to quantity as well as quality, for a small meal will often remain on the stomach while a larger one would be rejected; in proper exercise and careful attention to the condition of the skin (see page 46); in the clearing out of the *primæ viæ*, first by an emetic of ipecacuanha, and then by the due management of the bowels, for which we may prescribe the compound decoction of aloes with lime-water, the pills according to the formulæ given in the note,* or sulphur combined with magnesia and guaiacum.

* ℞ Pulv. Rad. Rhei.
    Aloes Socot.   āā ℈iss.
    Saponis Castil.
    Pulv. Calumb.   āā ℈i.
    M. Fiant Pilulæ xx.

Or

If the mucous follicles do not assume a more healthy action under this treatment, very small and highly diluted doses of creosote may be tried; and when the more urgent symptoms are overcome, very mild tonics, either bitters or chalybeates, are serviceable.

If the circumstances of the patient permit of his changing his place of abode, he should seek for a dry air, and should divide his time between a mountainous region in the summer and the seaside in winter.

There is yet another form of gastro-intestinal disturbance to which I would direct attention; I refer to *English cholera.* The patient is suddenly attacked, and almost always in the middle of the night, with vomiting and diarrhœa. The remains of the last meal are first brought up, and afterwards mucus mixed with bile. The diarrhœa is very severe, and is accompanied with violent colic, which is regarded by the patient as far the most urgent symptom. Occasionally I have found that there have been premonitory symptoms for a few days previously—a loss of appetite, thirst, and general discomfort—but these cases are comparatively rare.

The vomiting most commonly ceases spontaneously in a few hours, and almost always disappears before any very marked alteration has taken place in the diarrhœa.

This diarrhœa is sometimes very unmanageable, and merges closely on dysentery.

This is especially a summer disease. It can often be directly traced to the use of unripe fruit, or to a sudden chill, but sometimes we can only vaguely ascribe it to atmospheric causes.

Although the disease will usually terminate favourably if left to itself, medicine affords great relief. Where the vomiting is very severe,* nothing allays the irritability of the stomach so well as effervescing draughts of citrate of ammonia. The diarrhœa and colic are best relieved by a combination of three grains of calomel and half a grain of opium every four hours. If, as I have often observed, the

℞ Pil. Rhei. Comp.
  Pil. Galb. Comp.   āā ℈iss.
  M. Fiant Pilulæ xii.

The Pil. Scillæ Comp. may be advantageously substituted for the Pil. Galb. Comp. in cases where there is much dyspnœa. A couple of any of these pills will usually insure a proper action of the bowels. They may be taken before dinner or at bed-time.

* In these cases we must be especially careful, when the patients have suffered from old hernias.

INFLAMMATION OF THE STOMACH.   133

diarrhœa is succeeded by constipation, we must have recourse to castor oil.

In violent attacks of this nature it is requisite, especially in debilitated aged persons, to keep up the heat of the body. A hot bottle wrapped in flannel, applied to the feet, and sinapisms to the calves of the legs, are useful auxiliaries to more active treatment.

The gastritis of aged persons next claims our attention. I use this term for want of a better. It is an objectionable one because the stomach in old age seldom suffers from true inflammation.

Aged persons are often attacked with symptoms presenting all the characters of inflammation of the stomach, on the sudden retrocession of gout, or on the stoppage of hemorrhoidal or other discharges. We may term this *metastatic gastritis*. It is very dangerous, and in many points presents a resemblance to cases of acrid poisoning.

Gouty gastritis often begins with spasm. The burning sensation in the stomach is at first not continuous, but varies more or less with the pain in the joint which was originally affected. It subsequently becomes constant; the patient cannot bear the least pressure on the stomach; there is a tendency to vomiting, and the respiration is frequently much impeded. The smallest quantity of food is rejected in the course of one or two minutes, and the vomited matter has a very acid odour. There is urgent thirst, great general distress, and the pulse is quick and weak.

Our great object in these cases is to recall the gout to the parts originally affected.

The symptoms arising from the suppression of the hemorrhoidal flux are very similar, and here our leading object must be to re-establish the discharge.

But at the same time we must attempt to allay the undue irritability of the stomach. If there are distinct indications of true inflammation, we must, whatever the patient's age may be, apply leeches to the epigastrium, or to the anus. We must also apply emollient fomentations or cataplasms to the seat of pain, and administer sedatives, such as opium, and hydrocyanic acid. In these cases opium may be given very freely, and I have frequently seen excellent effects from the ordinary combination of that drug and calomel. There are few cases in which greater judgment is required, than in those we are describing. Notwithstanding the inflammatory symptoms I have often found it necessary simultaneously to administer powerful stimulants,—brandy, ammonia, and sulphuric ether.

It has never fallen to my lot to witness any severe cases of metastatic gastritis from the suppression of bleeding piles. The treatment I should adopt in such cases, would consist in leeches to the anus, and stimulating injections thrown into the rectum,—of course not omitting the internal remedies already mentioned.

There is a form of *chronic gastritis* common in advanced life, which proceeds to ulceration of the stomach, and finally to perforation, and to the fatal effusion of its contents into the peritoneal cavity.

The symptoms of this form of gastritis are by no means clear: and the affection is often unrecognised till the sudden pain dependent on the perforation, and the peritonitis that is at once set up, too clearly reveal the true nature of the antecedent symptoms. The patient complains for a long time of severe dyspeptic pains and of an indefinite feeling of discomfort over the upper part of the abdomen. Vomiting is a frequent symptom, and one often difficult to check. Melæna or hæmatemesis is not uncommon. The patient gradually wastes away, and not unfrequently dies from inanition and slow fever, before the ulceration has proceeded to actual perforation.

If perforation takes place, death usually ensues within twenty-four hours. The same morbid process may go on in other parts of the intestinal canal. The symptoms are then much less marked, and I have seen more than one case in which the patient did not feel that he required medical aid till perforation took place.

The treatment of ulcerative gastritis in old people is unfortunately too often unavailing. Leeches and counter-irritants must be occasionally applied over the seat of the pain; and the greatest attention must be paid to the diet; animal food and stimulating drinks must be totally prohibited, and the patient kept on the mildest forms of farinaceous food. Milk and lime-water will often remain on the stomach, and excite less uneasiness than any other form of nutriment. Bismuth and sulphate of iron are amongst the remedies that have been most advocated in these cases; but their efficacy is often doubtful.

Cancer of the stomach is essentially a disease of advanced life. Of seventy cases collected by Canstatt only fourteen occurred before the age of 40, and of the remaining fifty-six, no less than twenty-one occurred in persons between the ages of 60 and 70 years.*

* Of fifteen cases of cancer of the stomach and œsophagus, described by Alderson, none were under 40 years of age: there were three between 48 and 50; three between 50 and 60; seven between 60 and 70; and two between 70 and 80. See Alderson's *Practical Observations, &c.* London, 1847.

The course of the disease may be divided into three periods.

The first may be termed the dyspeptic period. The tongue is pale, the mouth usually clammy on waking, and the appetite variable. Digestion is slow and laborious; there is a sensation of weight and distention in the epigastric region, lasting for some hours after a meal, and frequently relieved by abundant eructations, which have often a very fetid odour. Water-brash is frequent, and constipation is generally present.

In the second stage the patient complains of frequent spasmodic pain in the stomach, and there is usually occasional vomiting. The previous sensation of discomfort yields to one of actual pain, which is sometimes described as of a gnawing, and sometimes of a lancinating character. The pain, vomiting, eructations, and constipation, gradually increase, and by careful examination a tumour may often be detected at, or near, the seat of the pain. If it is seated at the pylorus, or great curvature, it is generally easy of detection. When it is seated on the lesser curvature, or at the cardiac extremity, it is by no means so easy of discovery. I have sometimes observed the eructations accompanied by intense heartburn.

The third stage presents the above symptoms in an aggravated state. The patient has become extremely emaciated. A nodular hard tumour is perceptible somewhere between the ensiform cartilage and the umbilicus. Attacks of diarrhœa frequently alternate with obstinate constipation. Every thing that is swallowed gives rise to vomiting. The skin, which in the second stage begins to be affected, now assumes the well-known tint characteristic of organic disease. The pulse can hardly be felt, and the patient ultimately sinks into a state of perfect marasmus.

Such are the most striking symptoms of cancer of the stomach. They vary, however, in many cases. Epigastric pain may continue absent throughout the whole course of the disease, and a similar remark applies to nausea and vomiting. Cases are even recorded in which the malady has run a totally latent course; and death ensuing from the result of accident, or of some independent disease, the stomach has been found in an advanced stage of cancer.

In regard to the treatment of this affection, we can scarcely hope that it will be more than palliative. Cases are, however, recorded in which the disease is stated to have disappeared after the prolonged use of conium; and there is little doubt that it is the most efficacious drug, with which we are yet acquainted, in the treatment of this distressing malady. Those who have used this medicine most extensively, advise that the extract should be employed, beginning with one-grain doses, two or times a-day, and increasing the dose, till the poisonous influence of the drug begins slightly to manifest itself. Dr. Walsh, in his admirable Monograph on Cancer, states that the only benefit he has derived from its administration has been the alleviation of pain and irritability, but Dr. Bayle in his summary of the recorded experience on the subject, finds that of 341 cases of cancer generally (not merely of the stomach) treated with conium, 46 were cured, 28 benefited, and in 267 instances the drug failed to produce any beneficial effect.

Palliation is more frequently effected by medicines that act on the nervous system, than by those used to counteract inflammatory action. Dr. Walsh recommends a combination of trisnitrate of bismuth with the extracts of hop, stramonium, and conium; and it is from this class of medicines that I have invariably seen the greatest benefit result. Whenever much pain is experienced in the epigastric region, I prescribe a belladonna plaster, and I have found this afford far more relief than any form of counter-irritant. When there is much tenderness on pressure, the application of the plaster may be preceded by that of a few leeches.

The sensation of pain must be allayed by opiates, of which an excellent form is the bimeconate of morphia, or if they seem to increase the constipation that is generally present, by the cannabis indica.

We are often called upon to relieve the flatus and vomiting in these cases; and it unfortunately happens that those medicines which relieve the former symptom usually, if persisted in, increase the irritation of the stomach. I believe that a drop or two of cajeput oil on sugar, as recommended in page 126, is one of the least hurtful carminatives. Vomiting may often be relieved by effervescing draughts of citrate of potash or soda, containing a couple of drops of hydrocyanic acid. In the treatment of the constipation, we must carefully avoid all drastic purgatives. If we cannot succeed in regulating the bowels by laxative medicines, we must have recourse to injections.

I must not conclude this subject without a remark upon the diet in cases of this nature. It is of the greatest importance that the quantity of food taken at each meal be small, that it be thoroughly masticated, and that the meal times be strictly preserved. All highly seasoned dishes, salted meat, and pickles should be avoided; and in most cases, a diet consisting in a great measure of milk, is best borne.

Whilst however some patients find that any deviation from a milk or farinaceous diet excites great discomfort, others find that they can more easily digest animal food. This is a point on which the patient may usually be allowed to judge for himself. It is a point of great importance in these cases not to swallow the food at a high temperature.

SECTION II.

Diseases of the Rectum—Congestion—Its Terminations and Causes—Hemorrhage —Danger of checking it—Treatment—Tumours—Their Treatment—Mucous Discharge from the Anus—Inflammation of the Rectum—Itching of the Anus— Stricture of the Rectum—Abscess near the Rectum—Paralysis of the Sphincter Ani.

WE proceed to notice certain affections of the lower portion of the intestinal canal—*the rectum*.

Amongst these we shall first offer a few remarks on *congestion of the rectum*,* a disease which although not exclusively restricted to advanced age, is very frequent in the earlier stages of declining life.

This congestion is generally manifested by a sense of weight and fulness in the rectum and perineum. The following symptoms, or some of them, are usually present: rigors, rigidity, and occasional spasm of the extremities, pallor, dinginess of the skin beneath the eyes, cold and dry skin, weight and pain in the forehead, vertigo, dryness of the fauces, white tongue, vomiting, temporary augmentation of the liver, flatulence, pain in the abdomen, constipation, scanty and colourless urine, increased velocity and hardness of the pulse, percordial anxiety, palpitation, syncope, hurried respiration, a feeling of weight in the loins, hips, and groins, dull throbbing pain in the rectum, attended with a sense of increased heat, tenesmus, mucous discharge, and occasional darting sensations, resembling those of electricity, itching of the anus, and finally, painful, difficult and frequent micturition.

This abnormal distention of the vessels of the rectum either subsides in a few days or gives rise to hemorrhage, the formation of tumours at the anus, or inflammation.

* In the description of this affection, I have freely availed myself of Bushe's *Treatise on the Rectum, &c.*

The causes of this affection are various. I shall mention the most important of them.

The structure of the part seems to predispose to the disease. "The absence of valves in the veins, together with the contraction of the muscular coat of the rectum, prevents the free ascent of the blood, and thus gives rise to sanguineous congestion of this intestine."

Towards the termination of mature and the commencement of advancing age, there seems to be a tendency to abdominal plethora, owing to the greater proportional development of the venous system, and to the comparative languor of the circulation. Moreover, in the female sex the cessation of the menstrual discharge usually (for a time at least) increases the plethoric state of the pelvic viscera.

Any morbid change impeding, either directly or secondarily, the pelvic circulation, as enlargement of the liver, spleen, or pancreas, or disease of the lungs, heart, or aorta may cause a hemorrhoidal tendency; so also may indurated and impacted fæces in the rectum, partly by compressing the hemorrhoidal veins, and partly by irritating the mucous membrane.

Stone in the bladder, stricture of the urethra, and an enlarged prostate, almost invariably excite a certain degree of congestion of the rectum.

Every thing directly stimulating the mucous membrane, as aloes and certain other purgatives, various articles of diet, ascarides, the acrid discharge in dysentery, &c., all act by directing an increased flow of blood to the rectum, in consequence of the irritation which they set up.

I need hardly add that sedentary habits strongly favour the accumulation of blood in the hemorrhoidal vessels, and that it is established beyond all doubt, that like the allied diseases of scrofula and gout, it is very frequently an hereditary disease. When the symptoms of congestion occur, the great aim of our treatment must be to relieve the over-loaded vessels of the rectum. The bowels should be freely opened with castor oil, leeches should then be applied to the anus, and after their removal a warm hip-bath is usually advisable. In those who have previously suffered from hemorrhage this treatment usually reproduces it, and relief is then almost instantaneously afforded; the symptoms however generally yield to the above remedies, whether a hemorrhoidal discharge be induced or not.

We have already observed that congestion of the rectum may give rise to hemorrhage, tumours (internal or external piles), or inflammation.

When *hemorrhage* occurs, it usually follows the passage of a motion. It generally ceases in a few days, but occasionally lasts for months. It sometimes assumes a periodic character. The loss of a very small quantity of blood often relieves the feeling of heat, weight, and tension around the anus, and likewise other of the symptoms recorded in page 137. The amount of blood commonly lost is various and almost invariably much overrated by the patient; it may be less than a drachm or it may amount, at one time, to several pints.*

Great caution is requisite in the treatment of this affection, for the sudden suppression of the sanguineous discharge is attended with great danger. I am acquainted with cases, in which it has caused death by brain-fever, apoplexy, and pulmonary hemorrhage, and have seen numerous instances in which great constitutional disturbance (not terminating fatally) has arisen from this source.

My own practice is not to interfere actively unless the loss of blood seems to render the patient weak and nervous. In fact I seldom do more than prescribe a sufficient quantity of confection of senna, with a little sulphur or bitartrate of potash, to insure a proper action of the bowels. If, however, I deem it advisable to check the discharge, I have recourse to the confection of black pepper, always taking care to warn the patient that he must not expect any immediate apparent relief from its use. I may take this opportunity of remarking that if an objection is made on the part of the patient, to take medicine in this form—and many persons, I know, experience great trouble in swallowing electuaries—the difficulty is easily got over, by ordering that each dose before being swallowed should be enveloped in a small piece of moistened rice-paper. The taste is thus concealed, the adhesiveness to the tongue prevented, and a draught of water carries the little parcel safely down the œsophagus.

When there seems to be a relaxed condition of the mucous mem-

---

* Montegre in his *Traité analytique de toutes les Affections Hemorrhoidales*, has collected many of the medical wonders, recorded by early writers in connection with this subject. We have "the case of a tailor, who lost as much as ten pounds of blood at a time. This man was nevertheless vigorous and of a jovial character." Smetius relates the case of a man forty years of age, who passed per anum, at least thirty pounds of blood, in two or three days. He was cured by *a tonic plaster!* Finally, Pezold speaks of a Saxon chevalier who in one attack lost sixty pounds of blood. This is about double the quantity that the Saxon chevalier possessed in his whole body.

brane generally, I have found small doses of oil of turpentine (ten drops three times a-day) of much service. In cases that do not yield to the above remedies, gallic acid or matico might prove successful. I have however no personal experience of their use in these cases.

When we find that the patient is much exhausted by a prolonged discharge, we may advantageously prescribe an acid solution of quinine, and sometimes even mild ferruginous preparations, with much advantage. For those who are strong enough to bear it, sea bathing is also highly serviceable.

Cold or astringent injections must be prescribed in advanced life with extreme caution.

The bleeding in many cases arises from tumours, which we now proceed to notice as another consequence of congestion.

These *tumours* may be arranged in two classes, according as they are situated within, or immediately without the anus. They are both of them the result of repeated attacks of congestion.

Those within the anus vary in number and size, and when large are usually prolapsed, whenever the bowels are moved. They are of a dark red colour, and when prolapsed, they become perfectly livid, owing to the strangulation produced by the action of the sphincter.

When they are small they give rise to a sensation of heat and itching, but as they become larger they produce a feeling of weight and distention in the lower extremity of the rectum, and as I have already remarked, are prolapsed after every motion. For a time the muscular action of the sphincter seems to replace them, but it often happens, that after a certain period this muscle becomes partially relaxed, and the tumours, in descending, draw along with them a portion of the adjacent mucous membrane, and it becomes necessary to replace the protruded parts by the hand. Many persons suffering in this manner, are compelled to postpone the evacuation of the bowels to the period of their retiring for the night, in consequence of the time required to replace the protrusion, and the difficulty of effecting it in any other than the horizontal position. When these tumours occur in cases of hemorrhoidal discharge, it is almost invariably from them, and not from the adjacent mucous membrane, that the blood is effused.

These tumours are very liable to inflammatory attacks, which sometimes give rise to small abscesses.

The only affections for which they can be mistaken are chronic prolapsus of the mucous membrane, and polypi.

The second class of tumours—those, namely, which are situated without the anus—are formed of extravasated blood inclosed in a cyst, and covered by a few fibres of the sphincter and by the delicate skin of the verge of the anus. They seldom attain to any great size, and the principal symptoms they give rise to, are a sensation of itching, and fulness about the lower part of the rectum and the anus.

Although this class of affections is popularly regarded as belonging to surgery rather than to medicine, there is no doubt that by careful management and purely medical treatment, surgical interference may often be altogether dispensed with.

Whether the tumours be external or internal, the anus should be kept scrupulously clean. For this purpose a lather of common yellow soap and water should be applied to the part after each action of the bowels, and before the piles (if they are prolapsed) are returned. This application is serviceable in two ways : (1) it completely removes any remains of excrementitious matter ; and (2) it acts as an astringent. Amongst the most important local applications we may mention gall-nuts applied externally as an ointment, or internally as a suppository. If the tumours are very painful, a little opium may be added, and if there is spasm of the sphincter, some extract of belladonna may be associated with the galls. Mild astringent injections may be tried.* A steel bougie passed a few inches into the rectum, and retained in that position for half an hour, is often of considerable service. It should be inserted every evening, and may be medicated according to the circumstances of the case. The bowels must be regulated by the means described in page 139.

If the tumours become inflamed, leeches, and, afterwards, tepid poultices or warm-water dressing, should be applied to the surrounding parts. If the tenesmus which commonly accompanies this condition of the tumours, does not yield to this treatment, relief is usually afforded by cupping over the sacrum, and by small but repeated doses of ipecacuanha.

Many persons who suffer from these tumours complain of a colourless mucous discharge from the anus. It varies considerably in its

---

* When there are no very marked contra-indications—as for instance spasm, or very severe pain—thirty grains of sulphate of zinc dissolved in half a pint of water may be thrown into the rectum after each daily evacuation of the bowels.

appearance in different cases; in some instances resembling thin gum water, whilst in others it approximates in its appearance to the white of egg. In the former case it exudes slightly from the anus, in the latter it is commonly passed at stool. There is usually considerable debility in these cases, and the most successful treatment consists in the administration of mild stomachic aperients, followed by the use of quinine and citrate of iron. Cold bathing and chalybeate or sulphureous mineral waters are often highly serviceable, but they must be prescribed with caution. The internal use of the balsams and of turpentine is recommended in this affection; and I have certainly seen good effects from the latter.

The local application of astringents is sometimes necessary. This practice must however be attended with great caution on the part of the physician; as if we check the discharge too suddenly, we may give rise to disease in other organs.

The third result of congestion, namely, *inflammation of the rectum*, may arise from other causes than those connected with a purely hemorrhoidal tendency. We shall therefore in the following remarks consider it generally, whether it arises from the presence of foreign bodies, indurated excrements, or concretions, from repelled cutaneous eruptions, from the application of cold and wet, from surgical operations, from the action of drastic purgatives or acrid secretions, or from hemorrhoids, gout, or rheumatism.

This disease is characterized by a sense of fulness, weight, heat, and throbbing in the fundament, which is most severe in the sitting position. The action of the bowels is accompanied with intense pain, which lasts for a considerable time, and, from the contraction of the sphincter, assumes a spasmodic character. On introducing the finger into the rectum—a proceeding which gives rise to much suffering—the heat of the intestine is found to be considerably increased. The functions of the urinary organs are disturbed. There may be strangury or even retention of urine. These symptoms are usually relieved by the treatment advised for tenesmus. The inflammation sometimes extends to the colon, and occasionally the peritoneum is also affected.

The treatment in ordinary cases is straightforward enough. Tepid emollient enemata (of marsh-mallows, linseed, &c.) must be thrown into the rectum, great care being taken that the process is conducted with extreme gentleness. Leeches should be applied freely, and **often for some** days, around the anus, and after their removal the

ITCHING OF THE ANUS.

parts should be enveloped in warm opiated poultices. No solid food should be allowed, in consequence of the irritation induced by the passage of firm motions over the inflamed parts.

I believe that this is the most appropriate place to notice *the itching of the anus*, which is a very common source of complaint amongst aged persons. I prefer considering it here, to postponing to the chapter on Diseases of the Skin, because it generally, if not always, depends on the same causes as the affections described in the preceding pages. It occurs in two distinct forms, namely, with and without an apparent eruption. My own experience leads me to the belief that there are two varieties of eruption which accompany itching or *pruritus* of the anus. One is the *prurigo podicis* of dermatologists —a mere local limitation of prurigo; the other is a vesicular affection, which however is often (perhaps always) associated with true prurigo.

Whether there be an apparent eruption or not, the causes and treatment are much the same. The itching is usually most distressing on getting warm in bed, and often prevents sleep for several hours. From constant rubbing, the skin about the anus becomes thick, dense, and furrowed. These furrows diverge from the anus, and vary in number from six to ten, and in length from a quarter of an inch to an inch. Amongst the principal causes of this affection we may mention ascarides in the rectum, old hemorrhoidal tumours, the neglect of cleanly habits, irritation or congestion of the prostate gland, and a morbid state of the alvine secretions, especially perhaps of the mucous follicles of the rectum.

The treatment must depend on the cause producing the affection. If ascarides are present (and they are by no means so rare in advanced life as is usually supposed), they must be got rid of. If there are old hemorrhoidal tumours they must be removed. The state of the bowels must be duly regulated; and light, nutritious diet recommended. I generally find that a mixture of equal parts of castor-oil and oil of turpentine is the most serviceable purgative in these cases. After three or four doses of this medicine, we may replace it by confection of senna combined with a little bark and iron. When there is an eruption round the anus, Plummer's pills and sarsaparilla constitute the ordinary treatment: five or ten grains of the former, and a pint of the compound decoction of the latter, may be taken daily. Various local applications have been recommended. Dr. Bushe, whose experience in the diseases of this region of the body has been extensive, has found far more service from rubbing the surface lightly over with nitrate of silver, and then frequently washing the parts with soap and water, than from any of the lotions usually recommended in these cases. The introduction of a steel bougie, and its retention in the rectum for half an hour, will sometimes afford ease when the affection is very distressing.

I ought not to conclude this subject without a passing remark on the opinion expressed by the late Dr. Lettsom, that this pruriginous state of the anus prevented the occurrence of more serious diseases. Although I am deeply impressed with a conviction of the extreme danger of repressing the "peccant humours"—whether they show themselves in the form of gout, piles, ulcers, &c.—I must confess that I have not been deterred by the perusal of his cases, from attempting and effecting the cure of an affection which, although apparently trivial, is often so torturing as almost to drive the patient to madness.

Stricture of the rectum is an affection too frequently met with in advanced life to be passed over in silence. It may be considered anatomically as presenting two forms—in one there is hypertrophy with induration; and in the other malignant disease of some of the parts entering into the structure of the gut.

As I have already remarked, the anatomical structure of the rectum renders it a common seat of venous stagnation, and it is this stagnation that is the primary cause of the structural changes that are so common in this part.

At first there is merely slight induration. The patient suffers from constipation, the bowels often remaining unmoved for several days, although he feels a desire to go to stool. There is a sensation of discomfort which gradually grows to actual pain, accompanying the process of defecation, and there is a difficulty in expelling the contents of the rectum, which are either flattened or in the form of thin cylinders. Moreover there remains a sensation as if the rectum were not entirely emptied. If in this stage of the disease we examine the rectum either with the finger or with a speculum, we find that a few inches above the anus, the walls of the canal are indurated and nodular, or even resemble cartilage to the touch, and that we are often unable to pass the finger through the obstructed portion. If the diseased portion is higher than we can quite reach, the patient can often aid in the examination, by forcibly bearing down. The examination is usually attended with considerable pain.

After a time these parts become the seat of ulceration. The distress of the patient is now much increased. A fetid discharge, consisting of blood and sanies, escapes from the ulcerating surface, coming away in jets, sometimes forty or fifty times a-day, whenever the patient coughs or makes the least exertion. The bowels almost cease to act. The transverse and descending portions of the colon are loaded with fæces, and may be readily felt through the abdominal walls, while the rectum becomes so contracted that it is hardly possible to insert the finger. The patient wastes away, and hectic fever sets up. The abdomen becomes swollen and painful; and hiccup, vomiting and ileus usually close the scene.

If the ulceration becomes very extensive, and the sphincter becomes much implicated, all control over that muscle is lost, and in place of constipation we have the evacuations passed involuntarily. The bladder occasionally becomes involved in this destructive process, and peritonitis, from the escape of urine, is then the immediate cause of death.

As it is only in the first stage that we can at all hope to effect a cure, it is the imperative duty of the physician to insist on a thorough examination as soon as the patient mentions any symptoms in the least resembling those of this fearful disease. He must not be misled by the patient's assertion that he is merely suffering from piles, and that he has had piles before, for even supposing that to be the case, not only does their presence not exclude the occurrence of degeneration of the walls of the rectum, but they often lay the foundation for that affection.

Amongst other diseases that may, without a due examination, be mistaken for stricture, we may mention hypertrophy of the prostate gland and retroversion of the uterus.

Amongst the most striking symptoms we may mention constipation, with occasionally attacks of diarrhœa, there being in the course of the day from six to twelve evacuations of soft excrementitious matter or of mucus, frequently mixed with a little blood; when the motions are hard they give rise to burning and lancinating pains in the neighbourhood of the rectum; pain in the loins and sacral region, or in the glutæi and thighs is often a well-marked symptom. There is a sensation of itching within the anus, and sometimes a shooting pain extending from the rectum to the glans penis. Some persons complain most of the pain after sitting for any length of time, others when they first assume the erect position.

As the disease extends, the pain increases, and is often at its worst a few hours after meals; the abdomen becomes tympanitic, and there is a feeling of distention about the region of the sigmoid flexure, which partially disappears after an evacuation from the bowels.

As I have already remarked, it is only in the early stages—when the stricture depends on mere hypertrophy—that we can hope to be of much service. Many years however sometimes pass by, before the patient's health seems seriously affected, notwithstanding the constant constipation and the daily suffering he undergoes.

The general treatment consists in keeping the patient as much as possible in the recumbent position, and restricting him to a diet which though nutritious, contributes little, or scarcely at all, to the formation of fæces; we may allow him extract of flesh, strong soup, turtle, oysters, milk, eggs, jellies, arrow-root, sago, &c. The bowels must be regulated by injections of oil and gruel, unless the passage of the elastic tube through the stricture gives rise to much pain. In that case we must have recourse to the milder purgatives, as castor or olive oil, cream of tartar, manna, cassia pulp, and confection of senna. Local pain and irritation must be combated with anodyne suppositories or enemata, and hip-baths; sometimes however the pain is so agonising as to require the administration of opium or Indian hemp. When the pain is connected with inflammatory symptoms, leeches freely applied round the anus, are often serviceable.

The bougie, and the mode of using it, require a few remarks. The constitutional effects produced by passing a bougie into the rectum, vary extremely in different persons; in some cases sickness, pain in the abdomen and loins, and shivering, follow its introduction, whilst in others it seems to cause scarcely any irritation. Hence the frequency with which we can venture to pass it, and the time it may be allowed to remain, must vary. Whilst in some persons we may repeat the operation daily, and allow the bougie to remain in the bowel for an hour or more; in others once or twice a week will be as often as we dare use it, and then only for a short time.

It would be out of place in this volume to describe the method of passing the bougie. I would merely remark that the bladder should always be emptied, and, if possible, the rectum washed out with warm water, previously to the operation, and that for ordinary cases, the best instrument is a short one made of India rubber, which may be entirely passed within the sphincter, and withdrawn by a ribbon attached to its extremity. Dr. Bushe uses bougies three inches long, made of ebony, and mounted on a stalk of whalebone. With either of these instruments, the pain caused by the prolonged distention of the anus is avoided. Nothing is gained by the forcible passage of large bougies. The cure is to be effected by pressure, so applied as to favour absorption, not by mere mechanical dilatation.

Abscess near the rectum is a comparatively frequent disease in old people, and deserves to be noticed in this chapter. There are several anatomical conditions which render this a common affection—as for instance, the abundance of areolar (cellular) tissue around the lower part of the rectum, the depending position of the parts, the large number of veins, and the accumulation of blood in them in consequence of the distention of the gut with fæces.

The following is a sketch of a common form of abscess. The patient complains of rigors and considerable fever. The pulse is feeble and hard, the tongue white and furred, the thirst urgent, and the skin hot. Soon however (often before we can ascertain the seat of the suppuration) the pulse becomes weak and irregular, the face flushed, the eyes suffused, the teeth and lips covered with sordes, and the tongue dry and brown. There are extreme debility and prostration, and more or less stupor.

The patient complains of deep-seated pain by the side of the anus, where we may readily distinguish a hard spot, which soon spreads. The pain then assumes a burning character, and there is considerable tenesmus and often dysuria.

The patient must be kept in the horizontal position, and the bowels opened by mild purgatives, such as rhubarb and magnesia with manna, or confection of senna with bitartrate of potash. The patient generally requires nutritious diet, with beer and wine; and small doses of quinine and sulphuric acid are often serviceable.

The abscess should be freely opened as soon as fluctuation can be detected, and emollient cataplasms sedulously applied, both before and after the operation.

If there is much slough to come away, stimulating dressings of elemi ointment, or of castor oil and some of the balsams, will be necessary.

Paralysis of the rectum has been already noticed as one of the causes of constipation (see page 127).

Paralysis of the sphincter ani attends most diseases in which there is much loss of power in the brain or spinal cord. Some years ago I was consulted by a gentleman seventy years of age, residing in the country, whose principal grievances were entire loss of control over this muscle and severe neuralgia in the dorsum of one of the feet. As far as I could learn from my correspondence with him, there were no other symptoms indicative of disease of the great nervous centres. Under the use of a milk diet, very minute doses of strychnine in an aperient pill, and the repeated application of tartar-emetic ointment along the course of the lower portion of the spine, these distressing symptoms entirely disappeared in the course of a few weeks, and up to the present time (a period of more than five years) he has had no relapse.

SECTION III.

DISEASES OF THE LIVER.

Gall-stones—Senile Jaundice—Ascites—Connection between Hepatic Disease and Apoplexy.

I now proceed to notice some of the most important affections of the biliary apparatus in advanced life, and I shall commence with the subject of *gall-stones*.

Gall-stones are more frequently met with in old age than at any earlier period of life. Those who wish to make themselves acquainted with the physiological reasons for this fact, and with the history of these concretions generally, would do well to read the section of Vogel's *Pathological Anatomy of the Human Body*,* which treats of the *special relations of unorganised pathological epigeneses*.

There is I believe no pain—not excepting labour pain—more severe than that arising from the difficult passage or impaction of a gall-stone. The impaction may occur in the common duct, the hepatic duct, or in the systic duct, the pain in all cases being very similar; and indeed a pain of nearly the same character may arise from concretions distending the gall-bladder, but not escaping from it.

The pain is most intense in the right hypochondrium; it is usually described by patients as of a grinding character; it extends towards the stomach, and shoots through to the back. The patient can neither sit up nor lie down, but assumes a doubled up position, his hands usually pressing upon the most painful part of the abdomen. The skin

---

* Pp. 333-375 of the English translation.

becomes covered with a cold sweat; nausea, sickness (the vomited matter being intensely sour), and faintness often supervene; the pulse is slow and quiet, seldom exceeding 60 in the minute, and, from the intensity of the pain, and the prostration induced by it, sometimes is scarcely perceptible. In some cases no food or even drink can be retained on the stomach. Short but perfect intermissions usually occur, during which there is no pain even on pressure. These attacks are often preceded or accompanied by rigors.

In most cases, jaundice is, next to the pain, the most prominent symptom; when however the concretion is impacted in the cystic duct, or when the attack is dependent merely on the tension of the gall-bladder, this symptom is absent, or only slightly exhibited.

When the flow of bile into the duodenum is arrested, considerable general disturbance is set up. There is occasionally great itching of the skin, and an eruption resembling nettle-rash. The tongue has a yellowish tint; there is generally obstinate constipation; if the bowels are moved the motions are pale, clay or chalk-like, and often in the form of roundish nodules. The urine is of a dark colour, almost resembling porter. Such are the ordinary symptoms of an attack of gall-stones. It may last from a few minutes to many hours. Persons who have once suffered, are extremely liable to future attacks; and the duration of each successive fit is usually longer than that of its predecessor. Thus in old cases, the attack occasionally lasts for several days; it then frequently excites fever and inflammation of the liver or biliary passages. As the concretion enters the duodenum the pain suddenly ceases, leaving only a sensation of tenderness.

In treating this affection there are two points to be borne in mind. 1. We must do our best to facilitate the passage of the concretion, and ease the excruciating agony of the sufferer; and, 2. We must endeavour so to modify the system at large as to prevent any further formation of these concretions.

To afford present relief, the remedies usually adopted are, opium in various forms to allay the pain, sulphuric ether and opiates, a mixture of three parts of sulphuric ether with two of oil of turpentine, of which half a drachm may be taken three times a-day, in any appropriate vehicle, and alkaline drinks as recommended by Dr. Prout. He advises that large draughts of hot water containing one or two drachms of carbonate of soda to the pint, should be taken. The fact that the first few draughts are usually instantaneously rejected, affords no indication against the frequent repetition of the dose. A little laudanum or any other fluid preparation of opium may be combined with these draughts. Injections containing narcotics and fetid gum resins may be combined with the above means; and warm fomentations applied to the seat of pain.

With an agent like chloroform at our command the administration of opium in excessive doses may altogether be avoided. There are no cases where this anæsthetic agent may be more advantageously used. It must be given in such a manner as just to deaden the sensation of pain.

How are we to prevent the further formation of biliary concretions? For my own part, notwithstanding the opposition of many physicians to the habit, I like, if possible, to clear the gall-bladder from the pent up bile by one or two sharp mercurial purges. The bowels must be regulated with mild doses of rhubarb and sulphate of potash, to which a little taraxacum may be added; and the free action of the liver maintained by sulphate of manganese in ten-grain doses twice or thrice a-day. Alkaline medicines are then of much service. As the cholesterin—the fatty matter of which human gall-stones are chiefly formed—seems to be separated by the liver from the blood, and as the fatty matters of the blood are chiefly derived from the actual fat or fat-making substances taken as food, the diet should be carefully regulated. Plenty of exercise, moderated of course according to the strength of the patient, should be insisted on.

In the above remarks I have confined my attention to the ordinary course of the affection. Gall-stones occasionally make their way directly into the colon, or escape externally, or are brought up by vomiting, but these are rare cases. I have only to add that when the concretion has once made its way into the intestine, we must carefully examine the motions, to see that it is ejected from the system. The evacuations should be placed on a coarse sieve, and water should be poured with some force on them, so as to drive all the soft matter through the interstices. The concretion is then left on the sieve. If it does not speedily appear, purgative draughts and injections must be administered, as, if retained in the bowels, it is apt to form a nucleus for an intestinal concretion.

There is a peculiar form of *jaundice*, to which old persons are subject, and which has consequently received the name of *icterus senilis* or *senile jaundice*. It is preceded for some weeks or even for months by a feeling of pressure and general uneasiness in the pit of the stomach, often amounting to actual pain, and most perceptible a few (two to four) hours after taking food. In some cases shooting pains are felt, extending from the stomach to the right hypochondrium, during the whole process of digestion. The skin in the meantime presents nothing more than a cachectic appearance, which is however gradually replaced by a true jaundiced tint. The above symptoms at first intermit, leaving the patient in a state of comparative health for some weeks; the intermissions however gradually become shorter, and at last altogether disappear. The skin finally presents a dull blackish green tint. The urine is dark from the presence of bile-pigment, and deposits a copious sediment. The state of the intestinal excretions varies considerably; there may be extreme constipation, or there may be grayish clay-like motions, or finally these last may be intermixed with black, pitch-like bile. The pulse is very slow. The patient complains of a dull aching pain under the false ribs of the right side, which is increased by a deep inspiration. A careful manual examination will frequently detect a hardness or tumour, the exact seat or nature of which it is often difficult to ascertain. It may be situated in the liver, the pancreas, the spleen, or the omentum. There is a gradual loss of appetite, accompanied with nausea, and often with vomiting; the patient wastes away, hectic fever is set up, the feet and abdomen become dropsical, and the emaciation finally becomes extreme. During the last stage of the disease, we frequently find that nothing can be retained on the stomach, and the peculiar matter resembling coffee-grounds is vomited, which we may regard as affording pretty certain evidence that there is organic disease of the liver, gall-bladder, pancreas, or stomach. Death ensues from exhaustion with convulsions and delirium, or from coma.

It will be seen that I have thus classed, in a single category, all forms of jaundice depending on structural changes. The symptoms, in all cases, are pretty much the same, and I fear we must add that, generally speaking, the treatment is alike unavailing. While gall-stones are most common in the female sex, men are most frequently the subject of the present disease. It is most common in old spirit-drinkers, in hypochondriacs, and in those who have been liable to attacks of gout or of hemorrhoids; in fact, it seems closely connected with a plethoric and torpid condition of the portal circulation. A sedentary mode of living, the use of unwholesome and indigestible food, constipation, the suppression of natural or artificial discharges, and, above all, the perpetual struggle for mere existence, to which thousands in this metropolis* are subjected, are amongst the principal causes favouring this disease.

The course of this disease, or, more correctly speaking, of the diseases on which this symptom depends, is very slow. The patient may live for years, the pain in the hepatic region usually increasing. A perfect restoration to health is only possible where the jaundice depends on the impaction of a concretion, or on the pressure dependent on an accumulation of hardened fæces. Most of these cases terminate in dropsy and hectic fever, a few in apoplexy, and fewer still in intestinal hemorrhage.

The treatment is seldom more than palliative, for the structural changes giving rise to the jaundice, are usually beyond the resources of our art. Much may be done, in some cases, by a judicious regulation of the diet,† and the regular administration of mild laxatives‡ and anodynes. Diet-drinks, containing taraxacum, burdock, or sarsaparilla, combined with muriate of ammonia, liquor potassæ, or small doses of bichloride of mercury, have checked the progress of the disease for a time. The free inunction of iodide of lead ointment may be associated with the above internal remedies.

Dropsy of the abdomen, although like jaundice, a symptom of various morbid changes, demands a passing notice. There are several forms of abdominal dropsy common in advanced life. One of the

---

* There is undoubted evidence showing that no less than *fifty thousand* of our fellow creatures rise every morning in London, without knowing how to obtain the most ordinary subsistence for the day, or where to lay their heads the following night.

† The subject of jaundice recalls to my mind an apt but very singular illustration of the facility with which some persons, in attempting to philosophize, misuse facts. Cattle are said to be subject to biliary calculi, while they are stalled up during the winter, and to lose the complaint when they are turned out to the fresh spring pastures. Hence it was argued that *grass* was a good remedy for jaundice. Van Swieten tells us that he cured a poor man, aged sixty, who had suffered from jaundice for twelve years, by making him live upon grass for two years, except during that part of the winter when there was none to be got. " At first," says Van Swieten, " the man rather disliked this diet, but in time he was well satisfied, and could easily distinguish the best pastures. At last he became a general nuisance to the farmers, for they found he had such a large appetite that they drove him first from one field, and then from another, and he was obliged to eat his grass secretly. *He was, however, quite cured!"*

‡ Ox-gall is a good purgative in these cases, as it supplies, to a great degree, the place of the natural secretion. I frequently prescribe it in combination with rhubarb and aloes.

most common depends on a morbid condition of the portal circulation, and we may, therefore, term it *dropsy dependent on the portal system*. It is identical, or nearly so, with the *ascites venosus s. periodicus* of Schönlein.* It attacks almost exclusively persons between sixty and seventy years of age, who have suffered in earlier life from gout or hemorrhoids, but who no longer have attacks of acute gout or hemorrhoidal discharges to carry off the peccant matter—the *materies morbi*—from the system. The general reaction which was previously capable of throwing off this matter, is, however, now wanting; and we can trace its feeble remains in slight febrile reaction, and in irritation, and, perhaps, a slight eruption of the skin.

The stagnant and loaded state of the portal circulation, combined with the absence of sufficient reaction to eliminate the peccant matter, gives rise in course of time to dropsical effusions, which usually make their appearance in the generative organs, buttocks, loins, and thighs, before we can observe any œdema of the ankles. The urine becomes scanty, depositing a copious sediment of pink urates. Abdominal swelling is now perceptible, but at first is not constant. After existing for a few days, there is, perhaps, an increased action of the kidneys and skin, causing it to lessen or disappear for a short time. It soon, however, becomes temporarily persistent; that is to say, it lasts for a space of time varying from six or eight days to three or four weeks, or longer, when it usually disappears simultaneously with the occurrence of an abundant perspiration, and a copious sediment in the urine. The patient feels better—well, perhaps—for a time. But the attacks recur with almost unfailing certainty, and gradually become more and more aggravated, till at length there is confirmed ascites. This condition of the portal system often gives rise also to structural changes, which take a share in the production of the dropsy.

This form of dropsy is apparently nothing more than an anomalous form of gout dependent partly on the want of power in the system at an advanced period of life, and partly on external depressing influences, as deficient nourishment, exposure to cold and wet, excessive grief or anxiety, great loss of blood, &c.

The disease usually runs a very chronic course, and although by judicious treatment, we can often greatly prolong the intervals between the attacks, we can seldom hope to effect a perfect cure. The

---

* *Allgemeine und specielle Pathologie und Therapie*, vol. 3, p. 200.

appearance of a hemorrhoidal discharge is a highly favourable symptom, and the more perfect the crises by the skin and kidneys are, the longer succeeding intermission may we hope for.

Warm weather is essential to the well-being of patients with this disease, and in cold, damp weather the temperature of their rooms must be carefully regulated.

When there is much turgescence of the portal system, leeches must be applied to the anus and to the pit of the stomach, and we may attempt to establish a hemorrhoidal discharge by the internal administration of aloes, or by means of aloetic injections into the rectum.

How are we to get rid of the accumulated fluid? Schönlein has remarked, and I believe with much truth, that this must depend in a great measure on the *fons et origo mali;* in short, that a difference in treatment is required according as the patient has suffered previously from hemorrhoids or gout.

In the former case we must stimulate the intestinal mucous membrane to increased action; but, in so doing we must guard against employing weakening and depressing means. A pretty sharp purgative, consisting of aloes, colocynth, scammony, and jalap, should be administered every fourth or fifth day, and in the intervals the bowels must be kept slightly relaxed by confection of senna, sulphur, bitartrate of potash, &c. Diuretics and diaphoretics may also be administered in the intervals between the purgatives. As soon as nature, thus assisted by art, has thrown off the morbid accumulation, we must attempt to give tone to the system by tonics and a more nourishing diet.

With patients who have previously suffered from gout, we must adopt a very different course. Here we must trust to the kidneys and skin, and must prescribe Dover's powder, guaiacum, acetate of ammonia, sweet spirits of nitre, sulphureous waters, and sulphur baths.

In both varieties much depends on the subsequent general management of the patient—on his diet, exercise, due attention to temperature, &c.

Then there is the form termed *organic dropsy* by many writers. It is the dropsy dependent on (1) diseases of the liver (hypertrophy, atrophy, morbid deposits, &c.), (2) diseases of the spleen (generally hypertrophy), (3) of the stomach (carcinoma); and (4) the female generative organs (hypertrophy of the uterus, or degeneration of the ovaria). The name is a bad one, as the *organic dropsy* of the writers referred to does not include the dropsies depending on organic changes in the kidneys or heart.

It is needless to enter into the treatment of organic dropsy, as it is merely a symptom of a highly perilous alteration of structure of one of the abdominal viscera. I would only add that, as far as the removal of the fluid by paracentesis is concerned, I have more than once had occasion to regret that I have allowed the operation to be delayed to a stage at which little could be reasonably expected from any human aid.

The dropsies depending on cardiac or renal causes are duly noticed in the Chapters on the *Diseases of the Heart*, and *on the Genito-urinary Organs*.

The connection between *apoplexy* and *hepatic disease* has been long vaguely recognised. The attention of the profession has been lately re-directed to this subject by Mr. Corfe, who, in his " Semeiotics of Disease" has clearly shown how biliary congestion gives rise to coma and other symptoms that are usually called apoplectic ; and further how, when the liver is thoroughly relieved, these head-symptoms spontaneously disappear.

CHAPTER X.

DISEASES OF THE ORGANS OF CIRCULATION.

Functional Diseases of the Heart—Palpitation—Fainting—Neuralgia of the Heart—Organic Diseases of the Heart—Their Fatality—Alterations presented by the aged Heart—General Remarks on the Treatment of Organic Disease of the Heart—Dropsy from Disease of the Heart.

I have briefly alluded, in pp. 35-6, to the changes that the organs of circulation commonly undergo in advanced life. The statement that " the size of the heart and the thickness of its walls usually diminish with advancing years" is, I believe, strictly correct in itself, but the extreme frequency of changes in the aortic valves, in the coats of the aorta, and in the capillaries, giving the heart additional work to perform, renders a certain degree of hypertrophy remarkably common, and has led some of our best observers[*] to conclude that in

---

[*] On this subject the reader may consult Bizot's well-known memoir in the

the majority of cases the heart continues to increase to the end of life. An examination of the works referred to in the foot-note, will show that the heart in aged persons usually presents alterations in connection with the valves and orifices, which in earlier life would have been deemed indicative of serious disease.

My observations on heart diseases will be brief and somewhat discursive, because for the most part their treatment in old persons is much the same as in earlier life. I shall divide them into the *functional* and the *organic*.

Amongst the functional affections, or those which do not *necessarily* involve any organic change, I place palpitation, syncope or fainting, angina pectoris, and neuralgia of the heart.

Palpitation is by no means uncommon in old persons. Independently of the various forms of organic disease of the heart or large vessels, on which it may depend, or which it accompanies, it may arise from various morbid conditions of the chylopoietic viscera, as for instance from enlargement of the liver or spleen, from flatulence, or from any other manifestation of abdominal plethora. Closely connected with this condition is gout, and every practitioner must have observed how very frequently gouty persons suffer from this affection. The palpitations in this class of cases either precede an attack, and usually disappear when the gout manifests itself in its ordinary locality; or occur when the gout suddenly disappears from the part first affected; in the latter case they are the most severe and dangerous.

Too active exercise, as walking fast, running, ascending eminences, &c., is more likely to induce palpitation in old persons than during earlier life,[*] in consequence of the deteriorated condition of the heart and lungs; and when it is once excited, the circulation is a longer time in regaining its equilibrium.

Palpitation from functional disturbance is by no means so dangerous as that depending on changes in the heart's structure. To dis-

---

first volume of the *Mem. de la Soc. de Méd. Obs.*; the various memoirs of Dr. Clendinning; Hasse's *Pathological Anatomy of the Organs of Circulation and Respiration*, p. 157 (Swaine's Translation), Engel's *Entwurf einer pathologisch-anatomischen Propädeutik*, p. 77; Beau, *Etudes cliniques sur les maladies des Vieillards* (published in his own Journal, for Oct., 1843), and Neucourt, *De l'état du Cœur chez le Vieillard*, in the *Archives Gen. de Médicine*, Sept., 1843.

[*] Senac relates the case of an officer aged seventy-two, who ascended a high mountain with considerable activity. Palpitation and difficulty of breathing ensued, and he died in less than six hours.

tinguish between these varieties, we must avail ourselves of the aid afforded us by auscultation and percussion, choosing for the examination a time when there is a total or partial remission. We must, however, regard neither form too lightly, for old people liable to palpitation of the heart very often die suddenly, and without any marked precursory symptoms. In cases of pre-existing softening, attenuation, or adiposity of the heart, palpitations are apt to give rise to its laceration.

Palpitation is not a disease that we can treat; it is only a symptom of something wrong in the action or in the machinery of the heart. Hence the necessity of accurately ascertaining its origin, before we attempt to remove it.

From whatever cause it arises, perfect repose, both of body and mind, is imperative. Most persons find relief on lying down; others, however, and especially those who suffer most severely on waking, are easiest when in the sitting position or propped up. As over distention of the stomach often excites it, the diet should be carefully regulated.

General blood-letting usually gives considerable temporary relief, and this is almost to be regretted, because the practice is a bad one, and if often repeated may give rise to a degree of prostration that may even prove fatal. A few leeches may, however, often be applied with advantage over the cardiac region.

The external application of irritants is far preferable; turpentine fomentations, mustard poultices, and the immersion of the feet and legs in hot water, are serviceable during the urgency of the attack, and they should be followed up by tartar emetic or croton-oil ointments or embrocations, dry cupping, and the use of the flesh-brush; in other less urgent cases more benefit is derived from belladonna and other soothing plasters.

With respect to internal measures, when the palpitation seems to be simply nervous, digitalis in various forms of combination is the most popular remedy. Prussic acid and the salts of morphia are often useful in these cases. Attention must at the same time be paid to the action of the bowels and kidneys.

Although the infusion of digitalis acts freely on the kidneys, the tincture (the form most appropriate in these cases) often exerts no marked effect on those organs, unless combined with nitrate of potash, the alkaline carbonates, &c.

Sometimes nothing acts so effectually as a little muriate of morphia, scattered over a small blistered surface on the cardiac region.

There is an allied class of cases, hard to describe clearly, in which the above remedies aggravate rather than relieve the symptoms, and in which the most benefit is derived from the fetid gum-resins, valerianate of zinc, and nitrate of silver.

When the affection is connected with gout, we must endeavour to induce or recall the attack in the joint usually suffering. The bowels must be carefully regulated, and one of the best medicines for this purpose is Murray's fluid effervescing preparation of magnesia. When the fit is very violent, and attended with the peculiar anxiety and distress which are occasionally observed, an opiate administered in a couple of ounces of the solution of camphor will afford considerable relief.

There is a peculiar form of palpitation depending simply on weakness of the heart's action. In place of the ordinary impulse we perceive a mere flutter or tremor; the pulse is weak and irregular, and seems to disappear on pressure; and the body generally presents the ordinary signs of debility. In these cases our main object is to invigorate the patient. We must recommend a highly nourishing diet, a moderate allowance of wine, and a residence in a dry, bracing locality, whilst the strictly medical treatment must consist in the administration of stimulants, as ammonia or ether, of quinine and the other vegetable bitters, of the mineral acids, and subsequently of the milder chalybeate waters.

Syncope or *fainting* is next to be considered—an affection depending conjointly on the heart and brain. Its ordinary duration is from a few seconds to a few minutes, but occasionally it lasts for hours and even days. Although comparatively free from danger when simply dependent on the reduced power of the cardiac nerves, it must be regarded as a very formidable symptom, when accompanying organic disease. A slight over-exertion often brings it on in old debilitated persons; thus I have known it on several occasions induced by straining at the water-closet. A similar effect is produced by postponing the taking of food much beyond the ordinary time; thus an old person accustomed to dine at two or three o'clock, will find that at five or six o'clock his appetite is completely gone, and he will feel sick and faint, unless he has taken any intermediate refreshment.

The first thing to be done in reference to treatment is to loosen the neck-handkerchief, stays, or any other portion of the clothes that may in any way be impeding the freedom of the circulation or the action of the respiratory organs, to sprinkle the face and chest with cold water, and to place the patient in such a position as, if possible, to expose him to a free current of air. He should be kept, till he revives, in the horizontal position, smelling salts and aromatic vinegar should be applied to the nostrils, and eau de Cologne rubbed on the temples, face, and chest; and as soon as he is able to swallow—but on no account sooner—he should have half a glass of wine. If the above means are insufficient to restore animation, we must have recourse to the galvano-magnetic current, which is the most powerful stimulant in our possession.

In debilitated persons who have a tendency to fainting fits, it is a point of importance to prevent the actual attack. This may often be managed by judicious dietetic arrangements.

Angina pectoris is essentially a disease of declining life, since of 84 cases collected by Dr. Forbes in his admirable monograph on this subject, 72 were above the age of 50. It is a comparatively rare disease, and I have not seen a sufficient number of cases to justify me in offering any remarks on it.

Neuralgia of the heart is an affection in some degree resembling angina pectoris, but far milder in degree. I am frequently consulted by persons about sixty years of age for this disease. They complain of a severe shooting pain, coming on equally whether they are quiet or moving, and extending from the region of the heart to the shoulder-blade; there is generally more or less irregularity in the heart's action; and flatulence and other symptoms of dyspepsia are usually present. The application of a belladonna plaster or of the tincture of aconite* to the cardiac region, and a little attention to the digestive organs, usually relieve the pain for the time. When the digestive organs again become disordered the pain is liable to return.

I shall offer very few remarks, and those only of a general nature, on the *organic diseases* of the heart.

I have shown, in page 66, that out of the 53,048 persons who, during the five years extending from January 1843 to December 1847, died in the metropolis at the age of sixty or upwards, the deaths from

---

* Equal parts of tincture of aconite and soap-liniment form a good embrocation in these cases. In all forms of heart disease, accompanied with pain or with excessive action, the internal use of the tincture is deserving of trial. Three minims may be given four times a-day. See Dr. Fleming's excellent Essay on the *Aconitum Napellus*. Lond. 1845.

diseases of the circulating system amounted to 2841, or about 5·35 per cent. Of these 2841 deaths, 2722 (or very nearly 96 per cent.) are ascribed to diseases of the heart, 72 to pericarditis, and 47 to aneurism. As the diseases we have hitherto considered are, with the exception of angina pectoris, comparatively seldom fatal, the great majority of the 2722 deaths may be fairly ascribed to organic disease.

There are a few points connected with the anatomy of the aged heart that seem to require notice, as being connected with certain of its peculiarities of action. The orifices of the heart become larger in advanced life. "The progressive enlargement of the two auriculo-ventricular orifices is tolerably uniform; that of the two arterial mouths differs; both increase equally until the meridian of life, but the aortic orifice enlarges more rapidly in advanced age than that of the pulmonary artery, so that in old persons the latter is even narrower than the aorta."* This enlargement of the orifices is undoubtedly dependent on the prolongation of the heart's action, and probably takes a part in the intermittence and irregularity† of its beats, which are so commonly observed at this period of life. The valves are usually more or less changed in advanced life, and I have had, on two or three occasions, satisfactory evidence of very considerable insufficiency of the aortic valves, without their having given rise to any corresponding symptoms during life.

The following remarks apply to the treatment of all the forms of organic change in this organ.

We must not be induced by the apparent urgency of the symptoms to open a vein without well weighing the danger. Those who have seen the alarming syncope—the temporary death—that in certain states of the heart may be produced in old persons by a slight venesection, will hardly require this caution. The livor of the face and lips may be intense, and the orthopnœa almost insupportable, and yet we may relieve the patient as effectually, although perhaps not so rapidly, by stimulating the circulation in the skin by friction, liniments, &c., by immersing the legs and feet, and if necessary the hands and arms, in hot water to which mustard or nitro-muriatic acid has been added, by the administration of musk and camphor, and by

---

* Hasse, *op. cit.*, p. 157.

† On examining the bodies of persons who during life have suffered from very irregular action of the heart, we often find firm clots of fibrin entangled in the *columnæ carneæ*. Did they exist during life, and give rise to these symptoms?

tincture of assafœtida given with a little gruel as an injection. If these means are not sufficient, a few leeches applied to the cardiac region, or a cupping-glass between the shoulders, are usually as effective in allaying the urgent symptoms as venesection would be, and are unaccompanied by danger.

In incipient dropsy from heart disease, digitalis, properly administered, will often do away with the apparent necessity for blood-letting. In advanced life it is usually advisable to combine it with bark or steel. Is digitalis of service in heart-disease when it exerts no action on the kidneys?

A great deal of our success in treating organic diseases of the heart consists in the proper management of the organs of excretion, especially of the kidneys, and of the bronchial tubes, and in a due and very strict regulation of the diet. All influences, whether corporeal or psychical, which disturb the regularity of the circulation, must be most carefully avoided. There are, I believe, no cases in which the patient will not find relief from sponging the chest daily with cold water, and from the subsequent application of a rough towel and the flesh-brush.

I have a few remarks to make on *dropsy*, dependent on disease of the heart. Partial dropsical swellings are usually observed in the face, especially in the eyelids on waking, in the feet and ankles in the evening, and in the hands, for a considerable period before there is any decided effusion or accumulation of fluid in the chest or abdomen. As the effusion increases in the upper part of the body, the patient requires to lie with his head and neck in a more elevated position than usual; and on its further increasing and extending to the other closed cavities of the body, he cannot lie down at all. When the cardiac disease consists chiefly of dilatation of the cavities and attenuation of the walls, the effusion is of a passive kind, and lowering treatment of any kind is certain to hasten the fatal issue of the disease. When there is obstruction in the valves of the left side of the heart (and this is the side thus affected five times out of six), congestion of the lungs often comes on suddenly, and the patient dies suffocated. Dropsy, dependent on this lesion of the heart, is often singularly amenable to treatment for awhile, but it is almost certain to recur, and finally to wear out the patient.

Before treating a case of cardiac dropsy, we endeavour to ascertain from the rational and physical symptoms the nature and seat of the lesion on which it depends.

If there be dilatation of the cavities and attenuation of the walls, the treatment must be decidedly tonic. If we cannot hope to remove the lesions already existing, we may endeavour to prevent their aggravation; and our main object must be directed to promote the absorption of the accumulated fluid, and at the same time to keep up the strength of the patient. In these cases the combination of diuretics with bitter or tonic infusions, and with stimulants, will usually be found advantageous; thus, as I have already had occasion to remark, iron and digitalis often constitute a valuable combination.

When the dropsy depends on obstruction in the left side of the heart, the pulmonary congestion that is usually present and aggravates the dropsical symptoms demands more active treatment. Free depletion by cupping, and by hydragogue cathartics, such as elaterium and croton-oil, are here of far more service in the first instance than diuretics.

CHAPTER XI.

DISEASES OF THE URINARY AND GENERATIVE ORGANS.

SECTION I.

Retention of Urine—Its various Causes—(1) Paralysis of the Bladder—(2) Enlarged Prostate—(3) Inflammation of the Neck of the Bladder—(4) Spasm of the Bladder—Secondary Consequences of Retention of Urine—Chronic Inflammation of the Bladder, or Vesical Catarrh—Formation of Stone—Peculiar Affection of the Kidney—Incontinence of Urine—Irritability of the Bladder—Hæmaturia or Bloody Urine.

RETENTION of urine is a very common affection in advanced life, and may depend on several distinct causes, which we shall at once proceed to notice. It may arise from
1. Paralysis of the bladder.
2. Enlargement of the prostate gland, or other circumstances giving rise to stoppage of the urethra.
3. Inflammation of the neck of the bladder, or prostate gland.
4. Spasm of the bladder, especially of its neck.

1. Paralytic retention of urine often arises from injury or disease of the brain or spinal marrow; it likewise frequently occurs in cases of typhus fever, or when the system has received any very severe shock. It is, however, by no means rare for it to come on gradually without

any apparent cause, and, as far as we can see, without any other apparent change in the system at large. In the latter class of cases the disease advances slowly.

The patient observes that the urine is no longer discharged with the usual power, but that it tends to fall vertically, and with little force beyond that of gravity, from the extremity of the urethra. The necessity of frequently making water is urgently felt, and the act of micturition is only partially accomplished, and with much difficulty. This difficulty gradually increases; the bladder becomes distended; and when this distention has reached a certain point, the urine begins to escape involuntarily, in about the same proportion as it continues to be secreted by the kidneys. Hence patients are often much deceived regarding the nature of their case. They consult their physician for incontinence of urine, and believe that they have lost the power of retaining that excretion; and are usually much astonished to find that on the passage of the catheter, several pints are removed.

It might be supposed that this distention of the bladder would have given rise to very painful symptoms. Such, however, is not the case, for the same diminution of nervous power which causes this affection, also renders the bladder insensible to the stimulating effect that the urine ordinarily exerts on it.

This form of retention of urine is scarcely ever met with, except in persons of advanced age, or in those who have made themselves prematurely old by a dissipated life, sexual abuses and diseases, and debilitating influences generally. I have already alluded (see page 52) to the danger of retaining the urine for too long a period in the bladder, and allowing the wish to make water to pass by without gratifying it. This is a very frequent cause of retention of urine, especially in persons who lead a sedentary life.

In the prognosis of this affection we must be guided by its cause, extent, and duration, and likewise by the age of the patient.

The treatment of paralytic retention consists essentially in the use of the catheter at suitable intervals, while, at the same time, we must attempt by appropriate remedies to restore tone to the bladder.

To effect this object cold sponging or the douche to the pubic and peritoneal regions is often serviceable, and electricity is likewise to be employed. In the event of these failing, a blister may be applied to the sacrum.

The following case* affords a good illustration of the value of the galvano-magnetic current in these cases.

Charles Crean, aged about seventy, was quite unable to void urine, and it was accordingly drawn off with the catheter three times daily. His mind has been astray during nearly the whole of the past year. He has been affected with paralysis of the bladder for some weeks; it manifested itself suddenly during a paroxysm of mental aberration.

On the 8th of October a current was applied (under the direction of Dr. Stokes) from the sacrum to the pubis, and along the course of the abdominal muscles. On the 9th he voided naturally a few drops. The application was repeated, and on the 10th he passed about a wine-glassful, propelling it at first nearly two inches from the extremity of the urethra. The treatment was continued daily till the 13th, when it is reported that " the bladder is evidently regaining its tone fast," and the electricity was discontinued. By the 16th, that is to say, after six days' application of the current the catheter was no longer necessary.

As the reporter correctly observes, this is an important case, as illustrating the value of this form of treatment, because no other remedy was employed.

Amongst the internal remedies, I may mention the tinctures of cantharides and arnica, as those which possess the highest reputation in these cases; the former, if not given with extreme caution, is however a highly dangerous medicine. I have recently been led to use ergot of rye very extensively in this affection with the best results, and I feel assured, that it is much more to be depended on than either of the above tinctures. I was led to give it a trial from the well-marked effects it produced on the bladder in patients who were taking it for another affection.

The form I prefer is that of a very strong tincture, prepared exclusively for myself by Mr. Twinberrow, of Edward Street, with six ounces of the ergot to a pint of spirit.

A drachm of this tincture may be given three times a-day in an effervescing draught of citrate of ammonia.

2. Enlargement of the prostate gland is a very common cause of retention of urine in men of advanced life. This change seems an ordinary consequence of age rather than of disease. One of the high-

---

* Graves's *Clinical Medicine*, p. 440.

est authorities of the present day* observes in reference to this subject, that " when the hair becomes gray and scanty, when specks of earthy matter begin to be deposited in the tunics of the arteries, and when a white zone is formed at the margin of the cornea, at this same period the prostate gland usually, I might, perhaps, say invariably, becomes increased in size. This change in the condition of the prostate takes place slowly, and at first imperceptibly, and the term *chronic* enlargement is not improperly employed to distinguish it from inflammatory attacks, to which the prostate is liable in earlier life." Sir Astley Cooper even went so far as to regard this affection as a salutary process, when it produces partial retention, " for it prevents incontinence of urine, which in old people would almost constantly take place, were it not for this preventive. It makes the urine pass slower than natural, but this may be excused, when it is the means of preventing a continual wetting of the clothes."

This change seldom occurs before the age of forty years, unless in combination with stricture of the urethra.

The following are the ordinary symptoms of chronic enlargement of the prostate in its most severe form. The bladder becomes irritable, the patient being usually obliged to rise two or three times in the night, and having more frequent calls to make water during the day than he used to have; he likewise finds that the process of micturition is considerably prolonged. These symptoms increase so insidiously as often to attract no notice till some irregularity—a chill, a slight debauch, but most commonly sexual excitement—produces a sudden aggravation in the form of pain and extreme difficulty in making water, soon amounting to complete retention. These cases are graphically described by Sir Benjamin Brodie, in the work to which I have already referred. The repeated attempts to make water having failed, the patient naturally becomes alarmed. The efforts to relieve the bladder soon become independent of the action of the will, and the whole of the abdominal muscles are thrown into convulsive action.

The bladder may be felt like a hard tumour rising above the pubes, and is the seat of an indescribable feeling of discomfort and uneasiness; and unless relief is soon afforded, symptoms of general reaction are set up, the pulse becomes hard and quick, the face flushed, the skin hot, and the tongue covered with a white fur. Exhaustion

---

* See Brodie's *Lectures on the Diseases of the Urinary Organs.* Third Edition, p. 151.

of the nervous power soon ensues, and there is a comparative cessation of pain; the tongue becomes dry and black, and the patient sinks into a state of coma arising from the non-elimination of the urinary constituents from his blood.

This is the most terrible form of the affection, but with proper care it ought never to be allowed to gain this ascendancy.

The following are the symptoms of the milder form of the affection. The stream in which the urine is ejected becomes gradually slower, till finally the fluid drops perpendicularly from the urethra; moreover, the patient can seldom retain it for any length of time; and either complains that he is compelled to evacuate the bladder every hour or half hour, or even less, or else that he has lost all control over that organ, and that there is a continuous involuntary dribbling of the urine, especially when in bed. There is slight pain along the course of the urethra, and often a free discharge of prostatic fluid. The motions often present a flattened form, from the pressure the enlarged gland exerts on the rectum; for the same reason piles and *prolapsus ani* are of common occurrence, and there is usually a sensation about the lower intestine as if it were not wholly emptied. To confirm the diagnosis an examination by the rectum should be instituted, and a bougie passed.

In this affection we can seldom hope to effect a perfect cure. We are often doing much if we succeed in arresting its farther progress.

With regard to treatment, I may observe that, although we have not much hope of effecting a radical cure, we may do a great deal to alleviate the misery caused by this affection. Independently of the regular passage of the catheter, which in advanced cases is essential, we are entitled to hope for better results than have yet been obtained from local applications to the gland. Ointments containing iodine and iodide of potassium, may be applied to the prostatic portion of the urethra,* to the perineum, and in the form of suppositories.

The general treatment consists in the prescription of a few leeches occasionally to the perineum, of a horizontal position, of a light farinaceous diet, and of mild cooling laxatives, such as confection of senna with sulphur or bitartrate of potash. Amongst the special remedies in most repute, I may mention iodide of potassium with liquor potassæ, and muriate of ammonia. The local irritation is often most satisfactorily relieved by narcotic clysters and suppositories.

---

* Stafford's *Essay on the Treatment of some of the Affections of the Prostate Gland,* p. 18.

In cases where the changes in the gland are not very far advanced, the above means will usually prevent the most dreaded symptom—the retention of urine, and will often succeed in relieving that symptom when it has already supervened.

There is a form of enlarged prostate simply dependent on *varicosity of its vessels*. It generally comes on slowly in old men who have suffered from hemorrhoidal affections, who are of a costive habit of body, and combine good living with a sedentary existence. In these cases a difficulty is experienced in making water after violent exercise, after partaking of any stimulating food or drink, but especially after any venereal indulgence.

The enlarged prostate is felt on instituting an examination by the rectum, but it is free from pain, and the passage of the urine causes no pain to the urethra.

The treatment consists in the application of leeches to the perineum and in the due regulation of the bowels. Clysters of cold water, or of decoction of oak bark with alum, are recommended by Chelius. The use of the catheter is sometimes necessary, and the hemorrhage that is often excited by its passage affords much relief.

The retention depending on stoppage of the urine from other causes than an enlarged prostate, as for instance, from stones or clots of blood in the bladder, are comparatively rare, and require no special notice.

3. Retention of urine, depending on inflammation* of the urinary organs, must be treated by antiphlogistic remedies. Calomel and opium must be given internally, and leeches must be applied freely to the perineum. After their removal warm anodynes must be applied to the lower portion of the abdomen, and to the seat of the leech-bites. Clysters of starch and laudanum afford considerable relief. The patient may be permitted to take any mild mucilaginous drinks, such as gum-water, decoction of marsh-mallows, &c.

4. Spasm of the neck of the bladder is no unfrequent cause of retention of urine in advanced life. It is, however, most commonly a secondary affection connected with stone or some other morbid condition of the bladder or kidneys, with hemorrhoids, or with a gouty constitution. We often, however, find it connected with senile *anuria* (the diminished secretion of urine, so commonly observed in old per-

---

* The symptoms are here so marked from the very commencement, that I deem it unnecessary to refer to them. It must not be forgotten, that repressed gout and cutaneous disorders are often closely associated with this affection.

sons), or occurring after the use of irritating diuretics, such as cantharides, or induced by a chill. I have likewise known it to be produced by too long a voluntary retention of urine.

The only disease with which it can be confounded is inflammation of the bladder.

In these cases we must have recourse to the warm bath, or hot narcotic fomentations, and to the internal administration of camphor and opium. The latter may be given freely both by the mouth and the rectum. We sometimes find that the spasm yields more readily to the tincture of the muriate of iron (administered in doses of ten minims in a little gruel every quarter of an hour till nausea supervenes) than to any other remedy. When the spasm depends upon the patient having voluntarily retained his water too long, we should not wait long to try the above remedies, but proceed to use the catheter, which usually passes into the bladder more easily when smeared with a little extract of belladonna.

I have nothing further to add regarding retention of urine in reference to its causes or treatment; it is necessary, however, to make a few remarks on some of its consequences as shown in the bladder and kidneys.

1. In connection with enlarged prostate we are very likely to have *chronic inflammation of the bladder*, which, under these conditions, is liable to give rise to stone. The inflammation is excited in part by the constantly distended state of the bladder, and in part by the tension of the mucous membrane investing the swollen gland. The inflamed surface secretes a viscid ammoniacal mucus, which probably tends to keep up the irritation. As we cannot have a better opportunity of noticing chronic inflammation of the bladder, it should be observed, that although it is very often dependent on diseased prostate, it may arise from other causes, as long-standing stricture of the urethra, stone in the bladder, or disease of the kidney.

The patient has frequent and painful calls to make water, and there is often considerable pain while it is being discharged. The urine abounds in epithelial scales, and on cooling deposits a thick tenacious mucus, which is often slightly tinged with blood. After this state of things has gone on for some time, the urine develops a fetid ammoniacal odour on its discharge. If the disease extends to the structure of the kidneys, new and more severe symptoms show themselves. The patient has shivering fits, nausea, and vomiting; the pulse becomes weak and irregular, the extremities become cold, and the tongue brown; and thus he sinks and dies.

This is the disease known as *catarrh of the bladder*, and is so called in consequence of the enormous quantity of mucus discharged with the urine. The mucus has an alkaline reaction; and when it is present in excessive quantity, it communicates this reaction to the naturally acid urine, and causes the precipitation, in a solid form, of phosphate of lime, which had been previously retained in a state of solution, by the free, but now neutralized, acid of the urine. This is often the source of stone in the bladder.

The following may be laid down as the general principles of treatment. The patient must remain as much as possible in the horizontal position, in order to prevent the blood from gravitating in the bloodvessels of the part. Opium is a valuable remedy in these cases, and may be given either by the mouth or by the rectum. The other sedatives, as henbane, hops, and lettuce, are also serviceable. The bowels must be kept gently open by means of confection of senna or castor-oil. There are certain medicines that are regarded as specific remedies in this disease. Amongst them, I may especially mention the root of the *pareira brava*,* the *diosma crenata*, and the *uva ursi*. These, in the form of decoction or infusion, may be given in full doses combined with a little tincture of hyoscyamus; or when there is a deposition of the phosphates, with a few drops of nitric or muriatic acid. Turpentine, cubebs, and copaiva, are often valuable medicines in these cases, but they must be given in small doses, and their action must be carefully watched.

This is an affection in which injections into the bladder are strongly recommended by some writers, and objected to by others. They never do good until the more urgent symptoms are overcome, and then the injection of any tepid mucilaginous fluid or of decoction of poppies, is often very serviceable. When the symptoms are still further abated, and the mucus is no longer tinged with blood, we may venture to try the effect of a very weak injection of nitric acid, as for instance, ten minims of the dilute acid to two ounces of water; the

---

* I believe that the best form of administering the *pareira brava* is as a decoction, according to Brodie's directions. Take half an ounce of the root, add three pints of water; let it simmer gently near the fire till reduced to one pint. The patient is to drink from eight to twelve ounces of the decoction daily.

In prescribing the *diosma*, I combine the infusion and tincture. The *uva ursi* is comparatively seldom given.

bladder should be washed out with a little tepid water before injecting the acid solution, which should not be retained for more than half a minute.

2. The kidneys are liable to become diseased from enlarged prostate, or from any other cause mechanically impeding the free escape of the urine. I shall not enter into the consideration of the changes these organs may undergo; it is sufficient to remark, that if the renal disease is not far advanced, it frequently subsides spontaneously as soon as proper care is taken to prevent the further accumulation of urine in the bladder. If, on the contrary, the disease has made much progress, our prognosis must be comparatively unfavourable; we may, however, afford much relief by treating the case as if it were simply one of chronic inflammation. The strength of the patient must be sustained by a nutritious diet; and a little ale, porter, or wine, may usually be allowed with advantage. When there is much pain in the loins, mild counter-irritants are indicated.

Incontinence of urine, like retention, depends on various causes; amongst which I may especially mention chronic enlargement of the prostate, paralysis, either general or partial, injury to the neck of the bladder or urethra by the passage of a calculus, &c. In some of these cases it is, as I have already mentioned, associated with retention. It is a disease seldom susceptible of a perfect cure. When the affection is unconnected with enlarged prostate, we can in many cases do little more than limit the amount of fluid taken, and enforce regularity in the passing of the catheter, particularly before retiring to rest.

Various mechanical contrivances have been adopted for preventing the flow of urine, or for receiving it as it flows. This is a subject, however, into which we need not enter.

Irritability of the bladder is an affection from which few persons in advanced life are altogether exempt. It may be described as a frequent and often irresistible desire to make water, unconnected with inflammation, or with any organic changes of the bladder and prostate. It may arise from various causes, but, as far as my own experience goes, in by far the greater number of cases it is dependent on an altered condition of the urine, which acts almost like a foreign body in the bladder. For the treatment I must refer to the observations in Section III. Irritability of the bladder is sometimes induced by the habit of too frequent micturition. (See page 53.)

Hæmaturia, or hemorrhage from the urinary organs, is not a rare affection in advanced life: it may depend on a want of tone in the capillaries of the mucous lining of the bladder or kidneys; or it may arise from ulceration or the laceration caused by a concretion. In the former case the mineral acids, with or without quinine, the tincture of the muriate of iron, gallic acid, and acetate of lead, represent the class of medicines usually employed. Small doses of oil of turpentine (from ten to twenty minims) have been more successful in my hands than any of the above drugs; at the same time I usually order a few leeches to the perineum or anus.

Hæmaturia sometimes proceeds from the kidneys in persons of a gouty diathesis. In these cases, in addition to the above line of treatment, we may prescribe carbonate of soda after meals, and small doses of colchicum at bed-time.

When the hemorrhage depends on ulceration or laceration, it is often found to yield under the use of cold diluents with tincture of hyoscyamus, the patient being kept perfectly quiet in a horizontal position, and on low diet. If this system fails we must have recourse to some of the styptics just mentioned. It is unnecessary to refer to the danger of allowing clots of blood to remain in the bladder.

SECTION II.

On the Diseased Condition of the Kidneys, accompanied by Albuminous Urine.

I PROPOSE in this section to notice that form of disease of the kidney commonly known as *Bright's Disease*. With regard to the origin of this affection, Dr. Prout observes, that about the age of forty, and particularly afterwards, many causes often co-operate to induce a certain change of condition in the kidneys, some of which may be considered as incidental to age; whilst others are the natural consequence of long-continued habits unfavourable to health, but sanctioned by the usages of society; such as the daily use of a full and stimulating diet, the free use of wine, &c. Of all other causes, however, particularly in large towns, venereal affections and their remedies, lay the foundation of kidney diseases in every class of society more frequently than any other cause. Although, however, the effects of youthful excesses apparently subside for the time, they are too often felt in advanced life, when the vital powers become enfeebled, and thus contribute to render old age miserable. Another frequent source of kidney disease is exposure to cold. Amongst the causes predisposing to disease of the kidneys in advanced life, Dr. Prout especially mentions a gouty or rheumatic tendency, and the natural decay of the vital powers that then begins to show itself.

The most characteristic features of this disease are uneasiness or pain in the loins, or a general feeling of indescribable debility; a dry skin; a pallid appearance of the countenance; and if the affection has made any progress, a puffy appearance of the eyelids; disturbance of the functions of the abdominal or thoracic organs, not however sufficient to account for all the sensations of the patient; more or less tendency to drowsiness; and a rather scanty discharge of urine, with numerous calls to make water. On examining the urine chemically and microscopically, we can at once confirm the diagnosis which the above symptoms would induce us to form. This fluid is, as I have already remarked, commonly diminished (I have, however, occasionally seen it increased); in colour it is somewhat deeper than usual, but as the disease advances it becomes pale; it is usually acid; it is clear when passed, but becomes slightly turbid on cooling, and often deposits a copious sediment, the nature of which I have described in another work.* On the application of a gentle heat, the urine again becomes transparent, but on raising the heat to about $170°$, it a second time becomes turbid in consequence of the deposition of albumen.

I shall not enter into a description of the microscopic characters of this sediment, but I may take this opportunity to observe, that no practitioner should attempt to treat kidney diseases of any kind without making himself conversant with the microscopical and chemical characters of the urine and its deposits. Chemistry and the microscope, in the hands of those who know how to apply them, are as certain guides to the correct diagnosis of renal diseases, as the stethoscope is to that of diseases of the heart and lungs. From the simple microscopic observation of the minutest portion of the sediment in these cases, I have often been enabled to predict that this affection would turn out to be one of Bright's disease before a trace of albumen could be detected in the urine.

The patient may remain in the state which I have described for

---

* See Simon's *Animal Chemistry*, vol. ii. p. 235–6, and plate 3, fig. 31, where the fibrinous casts alluded to in the next page are described and figured. For a full account of the blood and urine in this disease, I must also refer to this work.

many months (possibly even for years), till an examination of the urine reveals the nature of the case, or until some incidental cause (most commonly a chill), aggravates the disease, and brings on a degree of anasarca, either local or general, too marked to escape the most ordinary attention.

We most commonly find that, in addition to the peculiarities already described, the urine is of a rather low specific gravity; and further, that as the disease advances, the quantity of albumen is often diminished to a singular degree. In the middle and final stages there is always a great diminution in the specific gravity of this secretion.

I remarked that, if the disease has made any progress, we might observe a puffy condition of the eyelids. It is in this region that we usually perceive the first indications of dropsy, and it is most obvious in the morning; puffiness of the feet and ankles is the next marked indication, but this is most perceptible in the evening.

This disease, when it occurs in persons past the middle period of life, is almost invariably associated with some form of well-marked thoracic affection. M. Rayer states that in seven-eighths of his cases he found chronic bronchitis grafted on it, and my own experience fully confirms this statement. Next in frequency I should place asthma, sometimes arising from emphysema, and sometimes the form which I have described as cachectic asthma. During the final stage of the disease œdema of the lungs is also most commonly present.

I am inclined to believe that the other complications described by writers on this disease—disorders of the digestive and cerebral organs, and of the vascular system—are less marked in advanced life than during the period of youth and maturity. Chronic rheumatism often co-exists with this disease, but is, I believe, only associated with it, in so far as both affections often arise from the same cause, namely, exposure to cold and wet.

The thoracic affections to which I have alluded are most commonly the actual cause of death; sometimes, however, obstinate diarrhœa, or coma, arising from the poisoned state of the blood, closes the scene.

It is difficult to lay down general rules for the treatment of this affection as it occurs in advanced life. Local or even general bloodletting is very requisite when the disease assumes an active form, and before it has advanced very far. The bowels should be kept gently open by castor oil, or by colocynth and henbane;* when there is a gouty tendency, small doses of colchicum may be advantageously combined with the purgative; while, if there is hepatic congestion, occasional doses of the milder mercurials are serviceable. Mercury must, however, be given with a very sparing hand in every case in which there is even a suspicion of renal disease. The saline diuretics, as the citrate, acetate, and nitrate of potash, may be combined with sweet spirits of nitre. Under this treatment, and with a due attention to diet, the urine often returns to its natural state, and the various symptoms disappear for a season.

There are few diseases in which a rigid attention to diet is of more importance than in these cases. I have, however, nothing to add on this point to the rules laid down in Chapter II., farther than to advise that sugar should be taken with extreme moderation, and that in most cases fermented liquors should be avoided. Soda water, with a little hock, or better still with hollands, constitutes a good drink for most patients of this class.

In the more confirmed cases we must somewhat modify the treatment. We must still regulate the bowels as before. Diaphoretics, as the citrate of ammonia with ipecacuanha wine, Dover's powder, tincture of guaiacum, &c., are often serviceable, more, probably, from their action on the kidneys than for any other reason. The dry condition of the skin is much relieved by vapour or ordinary warm baths. Dr. Prout advocates the use of the infusion of diosma with extract of sarsaparilla, and the establishment of an issue or seton over the region of the kidneys in these cases; and, except in patients of a very irritable habit of body, I have seen the disease checked by this means for a considerable time, and a condition of the kidney induced in which mild astringents and tonics may be given with advantage. The *pareira brava* may be given in the form recommended in page 169, and the citrate or tartrate of iron, in very moderate doses, is fre-

---

* The following formula is one that I often employ:

  ℞—Extracti Colocynthidis Comp. . ℈ij.
    Extracti Hyoscyami . . . ℈i.
    Pulv. Ipecacuanhæ . . . gr. vi.
    Saponis duri . . . . . gr. x.
    Ol. Caryoph. . . . . . m. iv.
 Misce. Fiant pilulæ xvi. quarum capiat duas pro dose.

In advanced life, and when the constitution is much impaired, the drastic purgatives—elaterium, croton oil, &c.—are seldom applicable in cases of renal dropsy.

quently serviceable. Very small doses of tincture of cantharides may sometimes be prescribed with advantage in these cases. The effects of this class of medicines must, however, be carefully observed. In prescribing iron or cantharides it is well to combine it with hyoscyamus or conium.

With regard to the general management of the patient, we must warn him against bodily over-exertion in every form. A gentle walk, when the weather is fine, constitutes the best exercise. Riding on a rough horse, or in a jolting carriage, is almost certain to aggravate the symptoms, and is apt to give rise to bloody urine. Flannel should be worn next to the skin, and every possible precaution taken against cold and wet. Whenever the circumstances of the patient permit of it, he should reside in a warm climate during the winter months.

The thoracic and other complications add much to the difficulty of treatment. The most frequent complication, chronic bronchitis, must be treated in accordance with the rules laid down in Chapter VII.

When the tendency to coma, in the last stage of the disease, becomes very strong, and there is a general depression of the nervous energy, the effect of large doses of musk is for a short time very striking.

SECTION III.

On the Diminished Secretion of Urine in Advanced Life.

IN persons advanced in life we often find it a subject of complaint that they pass very little water. Further observation shows us that these patients present various indications of an impure or cachectic state of the blood, and consequently of the system at large. Amongst the most common manifestations of this affection may be mentioned:—

1. Rheumatic pains in the limbs; they are often worst along the course of the sciatic nerve, and are most distressing when the patient gets warm in bed.

2. Affections of the skin and mucous membranes; *prurigo senilis* and, occasionally, *pemphigus* seem connected with this state of the system; the lips and eyelids become the seat of herpetic eruptions, which often assume a somewhat intractable character, and give rise to deep ulcerous sores. Ulcers are also often seen on the tongue.

The ankles become puffy, and unhealthy; and flabby ulcers with hard edges form on them. These ulcers are generally painful, and secrete a thin acrid fluid, which hardens on their surface into a thin, dark-coloured crust. The mucous membrane of the eye is irritated, *lippitudo senilis* is set up, or, in ordinary phraseology, the patient becomes blear-eyed. The mucous membrane of the air-tubes is affected in a somewhat similar manner, giving rise to the form of asthma, described in page 88.

3. Cerebral affections—the headache, vertigo, drowsiness, and other symptoms that are premonitory of apoplexy.

The urine passed in these cases is dark-coloured, and if not absolutely ammoniacal, has a strong tendency to become so. It frequently but not invariably, deposits a copious sediment of urates and mucus; and usually communicates a feeling of scalding to the urethra. This condition of the urine is a frequent cause of the irritability of the bladder, mentioned in page 170.

This irritation is occasionally so great as to give rise to an irresistible desire to empty the bladder every half or even quarter of an hour, when a few drops are passed with considerable straining. There is often pain in the lumbar region, and sometimes bloody urine. It usually gives rise to hypertrophy of the bladder.

The digestive organs are almost invariably implicated. An excess of acid is developed in the stomach, and gives rise to sour eructations, and occasionally to vomiting. The appetite is capricious, and there is usually considerable thirst, but the amount of imbibed fluid seems to have little effect on the scanty secretion of urine. The bowels are irregular in their action, but generally constipated. The skin is dry and rough.

The persons suffering from this affection are generally upwards of sixty years of age, and most commonly of the male sex. Amongst the causes giving rise to it may be mentioned a predisposition to gout or gravel, a want of attention to the state of the skin, improper food, and spirit-drinking.

Patients often experience much relief from a temporary augmentation of the urine, from a diarrhœa, or from a sweat. In fact, whether the effete matter is removed by the kidneys or the intestinal mucous membrane, or whether it is eliminated by the skin (and it sometimes happens that a fetid perspiration bursts out), there is always relief for a time.

The constant desire to make water, and the irritable state of the skin, are the two circumstances that cause the patient the most concern.

There are several points on which our prognosis must be based. We must found it on the age and apparent constitutional powers of the patient, and on the duration of the disease; on the state of the urinary organs; and especially on the condition of the skin.

The following are the leading indications of treatment. We must attempt to remove the acridity of the urine and of the fluids generally, by a rigid attention to diet, by the almost unlimited use of mild diluents, and by the administration of magnesia or the alkaline carbonates. The condition of the skin must be carefully looked to, and the rules laid down in page 46 strictly enforced. Vapour and sulphur baths may also be had recourse to; and sulphur, from its well-established action on the skin and mucous membranes, should be associated with the other medicines given to obviate the constipated state of the bowels.

Small doses of colchicum combined with an alkali have often a marked effect in augmenting the urinary secretion. If these fail, the stimulating diuretics, squills, turpentine, &c. must be tried.

Various means have been attempted with the view of relieving the irritation of the skin. What succeeds in one case often fails in another. The application of almond oil, after the body has been washed or bathed in tepid water, is sometimes beneficial. Opium is essential in this disease; a moderate opiate at or a little before bedtime will often allay the irritation of the skin and of the bladder, and induce a refreshing sleep.

I have so frequently pointed out the danger resulting from the too rapid healing of ulcers, discharging skin-diseases, &c. that I need not allude to the impropriety of attempting to cure them in this affection. They are often the patient's greatest safeguard.

SECTION IV.

On Urinary Deposits, Gravel, and Stone.

THE chemical characters of the urine and of the various forms of gravel are so fully discussed in my translation of Simon's *Animal Chemistry*, and in my Lectures *On Chemistry and the Microscope in relation to Practical Medicine,* that I shall not advert to them in this volume.

A certain quantity of uric acid (in a state of combination) exists, and is held in solution in healthy urine. There are, however, certain conditions which give rise to the deposition of this substance from the urine in a concrete form. This separation may occur either before the urine is discharged or afterwards ; it is only to the occurrence of the former that we can strictly apply the term *gravel;* we shall, however, notice both varieties in this section.

The researches of Dr. Prout have shown that uric acid deposits are more frequent in persons of comparatively advanced age than during the prime of manhood. About the age of forty or later, uric acid is apt to be deposited, at intervals, in much larger quantity than usual ; and persons who have never observed these deposits before, now notice them for the first time. This appearance is often preceded for a few days by sluggishness of the abdominal viscera, which is relieved by the occurrence of the sediment. The above state of things, says Dr. Prout, will continue, or at least occur, till old age ; but frequently about the age of sixty or seventy, sometimes before, another change takes place in the mode in which the uric acid is separated from the system. At this period of life, the urinary organs not only begin to participate in the general decay of the constitution, but are apt to be deranged from other causes, and more particularly to suffer from the delinquencies of early life. Frequently also they become organically diseased, and this produces a disposition in the system to secrete neutral urine, or even the earthy phosphates. Under these circumstances, where the urine had previously for years deposited the uric acid, chiefly in the state of crystals, the crystals will in a great measure disappear ; and in their place a great abundance of minute globules of uric acid of various sizes will be separated from the kidneys. In most of these cases there is a good deal of pain in the back, and irritation about the urinary organs. This is always a dangerous state of disease, both in consequence of the great risk of the formation of a calculus in the kidney or bladder, and likewise in consequence of the danger that there is of suddenly checking the elimination of uric acid (see page 53). The most frequent serious affection resulting from its suppression is apoplexy ; but heart-disease is likewise common. Dangerous palpitations and great irregularity of action may be induced by the abnormal stimulus of blood, containing a superabundance of this material (as also occurs in gout) ; and further, this acid enters largely into the concretions often found in the aortic valves, and at the commencement of the aorta.*

Amongst the causes of uric acid sediments, may be especially mentioned errors of diet, undue or insufficient exercise, atmospheric influences (cold and moisture), and, in short, every thing that deranges the process of assimilation, and diminishes the vital energies.

The diagnosis in all urinary deposits is sufficiently easy to those who are conversant with the application of the microscope and of chemistry. (See my fifth lecture in the *Medical Gazette*, for Oct. 8, 1847, in which the various forms of the crystals of uric acid and the urates are depicted.)

In reference to prognosis, Dr. Prout observes that amorphous uric sediments are of a less favourable character in proportion as they are whiter, or of a more pure pink colour. When pale-coloured, they generally denote a tendency to the phosphates; when of a pink colour, generally some organic or deeply-seated disease. In drawing our conclusions regarding these sediments, we must likewise take into consideration the constancy with which they are deposited, and their amount. Whilst the constant deposition of a large quantity of amorphous sediment is almost sure to terminate in an attack of gravel or calculus, an occasional deposition in small quantity is hardly deserving of notice, and is most probably only a consequence of some slight error in diet.

When the uric acid is deposited in a crystalline form, the danger is generally proportional to the rapidity with which it separates itself. There is always a risk of the formation of a calculus, especially in those cases where the crystals have a tendency to agglomerate. I have already mentioned that the free deposition of uric acid is often highly serviceable to the system; it must not, however, be forgotten, that in persons of shattered and diseased constitutions it is as frequently the forerunner of a general breaking up of the system.

There are no affections, perhaps, in which it is so difficult to lay down general laws of treatment as in those we are now considering.

---

* A concretion taken from the aorta, and analyzed by Landerer of Athens, was found to consist of:

Uric acid	14
Animal matter	6
Phosphate of lime	62
Carbonate of lime	16
Carbonate of magnesia	2

Buchner's *Repertorium*, 1847, vol. xlv. p. 60.

A due attention to diet and regimen is of paramount importance in these cases. In this respect the rules applicable in earlier life apply to advanced age. A certain amount of exercise is always to be recommended, and walking is the most suitable form in which it can be taken. Horse exercise is generally too violent, and often gives rise to hæmaturia, or inflammation of the kidney ; while carriage exercise, especially in cases of enlarged prostate, not unfrequently occasions a species of excitement that had better be avoided ; and further, is of comparatively little service, in consequence of its not involving any muscular motion.

Alkalies are the medicines almost universally prescribed in uric acid deposits. They are given (1) to check or prevent their continuance ; (2) to dissolve concretions already formed ; and (3), with reference to their peculiar alterative effects.

To administer alkalies with the view of preventing the deposition of uric acid, they should be given so as to neutralize the excess of acidity at the period of its development during the act of digestion. From ten to twenty grains of carbonate of potash, with two or three grains of nitrate of potash to allay the irritability of the stomach, if taken three or four hours after a meal, will generally be found sufficient. This powder may be taken in a wine-glassful of water; and, when the urine is scanty and high-coloured, we may add to each dose half a drachm of the *spirit. ether. nitric.*, or *spirit. junip. comp.*

I believe it to be an exceedingly dangerous practice to administer large and concentrated doses of the alkalies or their carbonates, with the view of dissolving concretions existing in the kidney or bladder. The only method by which we can hope safely to attain this object (and at best it is but a hope), is to prescribe small doses in a large quantity of pure water; and I am by no means certain whether the water itself is not the more serviceable agent of the two.

I have already mentioned that about the turning point of life, occurring in those who have misused their youth and early manhood, about the forty-fifth or fiftieth year, and in others at a later period, deposits of uric acid are of frequent occurrence. The treatment must here be conducted, not only with reference to the undue acidity developed by the stomach, but likewise with reference to the congested state of the abdominal viscera which is almost invariably associated with this period of life. The *decoct. aloes comp.* is a serviceable purgative in these cases, unless when there is a tendency to piles, and we may add to it an additional quantity of alkaline carbonate, or a little pure alkali. Muriate of ammonia is also a valuable medicine, and occasionally we must have recourse to mild mercurials. When the due action of the liver and of the colon is restored, the diuretics mentioned in the last page, combined with nitre, and very small doses of the alkaline carbonates, will be found sufficient for all ordinary cases, unless there be a calculus already formed in the kidney. It must be recollected that in advanced life, and especially when the prostate or bladder is affected, the urine is very prone to become alkaline. On this account the action of alkaline medicines must be watched with peculiar care at this period of life.

Uric acid being an effete matter which should be eliminated from the system, medicines are occasionally prescribed with the view of increasing its quantity in the urine. Colchicum, turpentine, and opium, acting probably in very different ways, all produce this effect. Much caution is required in the administration of medicines given with this view.

We occasionally meet with deposits of the *triple phosphate of magnesia and ammonia* (the *ammoniaco-magnesian phosphate*), and of amorpous *phosphate of lime*, or of a mixture of the two, in the urine of aged persons. These either depend on local causes, as for instance, on disease of the bladder (see page 168), or on constitutional disease. In the former case our attention must be directed to the diseased organ; in the latter the use of sedatives, tonics, and acids is indicated. Opium may be given in full doses with great advantage. As the general treatment is the same as in earlier life, I shall offer no further remarks on this class of deposits.

I have repeatedly alluded to the tendency that there exists to the formation of stone when much uric acid is being passed. It is unnecessary to enter into a description of the symptoms indicating the presence of a concretion in the kidney, or in its passage from the kidney to the bladder; and I shall confine myself to a few remarks on treatment. Our first point is to remove the congested state of the abdominal viscera. We must cup freely over the loins, give one or two sharp mercurial purges, and then keep the bowels open with some of the neutral salts, as for instance, the potassio-tartrate of soda. Having thus relieved the symptoms of congestion, we have merely to prescribe the same treatment as if the patient were passing uric acid gravel (see page 180). In this way concretions frequently escape with very little annoyance to the patient. Great relief is often afforded by the occasional use of turpentine, as before suggested.

When the actual descent of the concretion from the kidney commences, the pain is generally very severe. Free cupping over the loins, and the prolonged use of the hot bath (almost to fainting), constitute the ordinary treatment, whilst calomel and opium are prescribed internally. Copious injections of warm water relieve the pain, and in cases of prolonged and severe suffering chloroform may be administered with advantage.

If the passage of the concretion is very slow, diuretics and purgatives seem to be serviceable. If the stomach is very irritable, they should be taken in an effervescent state.

Whatever can enter the bladder by the ureters can, generally speaking, escape from it by the urethra. If, however, a renal concretion be not got rid of in this way, it is almost certain to form the nucleus of a calculus.

Statistical investigations have proved than in all classes of life persons of a middle age are less frequently affected with stone in the bladder than those who are younger or older. Those who have had the most extensive experience in this class of cases, concur in the belief that, while amongst the (so-called) lower classes calculus is most common in children, amongst the wealthier classes it is very seldom met with till after the age of fifty. I have already given sufficient reason why the latter should be the case; there is, however, another which should not be overlooked. With advancing years the greater or less enlargement of the prostate prevents the bladder from being completely emptied. A renal concretion has, under these circumstances, comparatively little chance of escape; and further, crystals of uric acid, or any thing else that can act as a nucleus, are very likely to constitute the foundation of a stone. The bladder is then, to use Brodie's illustration, like a chamber-pot that is never washed out, and the component parts of the urine are very likely to be deposited in it whenever there is any kind of nucleus to which they can adhere. There is also another connexion between an enlarged prostate and the production of stone (earthy phosphate), to which I have alluded in page 168.

The symptoms of a calculus in the bladder of an old man do not differ materially from those presented in earlier life: on the whole, they are perhaps less severe. We occasionally meet with cases in which calculi of uric acid have remained in the bladder for many years, without giving rise to much inconvenience, except slight irritation and hemorrhage after any violent exercise; and there seems reason to believe that in some cases an enlarged prostate diminishes the suffering of the patient by preventing the stone from coming in contact with the most irritable part of the bladder.

I shall confine my remarks on treatment to the consideration of those cases in which it is not desirable to remove the calculus from the bladder by surgical means. When we are assured that the concretion consists of uric acid, our first object must be to reduce, by the means mentioned in pp. 180–1, the congested state of the abdominal viscera that always accompanies this species of stone; and, secondly, not only to regulate the diet and regimen with the view of preventing the recurrence of such congestion, but at the same time so to modify the state of the urine by the administration of the alkaline carbonates, &c. as to prevent the further deposition of uric acid, without interfering with the functions of the stomach.

If the above means have failed in checking the progress of the case, or if a patient have neglected to apply for relief till the bladder has become seriously implicated, we must adopt another line of treatment. When, as is then generally the case, the urine has become alkaline and the phosphates are being deposited, we can seldom adopt more than palliative measures. Opiates must be freely given. I commonly use Squire's solution of bimeconate of morphia; it may be prescribed either alone or with other narcotics, as for instance, with hyoscyamus; and I have seen decided temporary advantage from conjoining it, as Dr. Prout suggests, with a small quantity of an alkali. If patients cannot bear any preparation of opium internally, it must be given in the form of clysters or suppositories. The constipation induced by the opium must be counteracted by castor-oil, or when this cannot be retained on the stomach, by mild purgative pills. Relief may be also sought, and for a time is usually obtained, by the warm-bath, warm fomentations, large warm poultices containing laudanum, &c. Dr. Prout speaks highly of the temporary relief produced by a lotion composed of *Liquor plumbi diacetatis dilutus* and tincture of opium, applied as hot as possible, by means of sponges, linen cloths, &c. to the perineum.

It hardly falls within my province to offer any remarks on the nature of the cases in which lithotomy should be recommended, or in which we should dissuade a patient from it. I may however observe that the highest surgical authorities assert that age should be no bar to the operation, unless the stone is very large, if the patient be active and have no other complaint. The common enlargement of the prostate gland, says Sir B. Brodie,* does not add to the danger of the operation, and in fact, it succeeds, on the whole, better in old men between seventy and eighty years of age, than in those who are ten or twenty years younger, although the former are likely to have a prostate of a larger size than the latter.

I have hitherto abstained from offering an opinion on the possibility of effecting the solution of stone in the bladder, but I should be unwilling to conclude this section without expressing my most decided conviction, that in nineteen cases out of twenty a surgical operation might be dispensed with. Why then do affections of this sort fall almost invariably under the hands of the surgeon and not of the physician? I believe that there are two reasons sufficient to account for this. One is, that surgeons have, with few exceptions, never advocated any means proposed for this disease, which did not in some form or other involve an operation; they have clung affectionately to lithotomy as one of the glories of pure surgery. The other is, that a patient who has suffered from the exquisite tortures of stone is likely to choose the means that promise the speediest relief. The surgeon can effect, in a few moments, as much as the physician can hope to do in as many weeks, or perhaps months. But does the patient consider the risk at which this almost instantaneous relief is afforded? I say nothing of the physical pain, for since the discovery of the anæsthetic properties of chloroform† the worst forms of human suffering have been annihilated; I refer merely to the danger attendant on the operation. Taking the data afforded by the Bristol and Norwich Tables, I find that of one hundred and twenty-four persons operated on between the age of 50 and 60, thirty-one, or one in four died; of sixty-one persons between the age of 60 and 70, twenty-seven, or one in two and a quarter died; while of ten persons between the age of 70 and 80, three, or one in three and a third died.

There are two means by which the solution of a stone in the bladder has been successfully effected, (1) by the agency of medicines

* The data given below scarcely bear out Brodie's statement.

† Very few of my readers can entertain the slightest conception of the course of patient investigation and of personal experiment (often of the most perilous nature, and attended with severe results), that led to the discovery referred to in the text—a discovery which, when the jealousies and heart-burnings of our own age have been forgotten, and posterity can calmly adjudicate on the claims of a past generation, will lead grateful humanity to associate the names of Simpson and of Jenner, as the two greatest benefactors of their race.

administered by the mouth ; and (2) by chemical agents thrown into the bladder.

It would be out of place to enter into this subject in the present volume. I will merely remark, that no unprejudiced person can read the cases narrated by Petit, Chevallier, Robiquet, and many other writers that I might mention, without arriving at the conclusion that calculi of uric acid, urate of ammonia, and mixed and triple phosphates, may, under favourable circumstances, be dissolved or disintegrated in the bladder by the free imbibition of natural or artificial waters containing alkaline bicarbonates. It is my intention at some future period to publish the evidence I have collected on this subject.

SECTION V.

Neuralgia dependent on a Morbid Condition of the Genito-urinary Organs—Abnormal Excitation or Diminution of the Sexual Feelings—Uterine Hemorrhage.

I ALLUDED to these neuralgic pains in page 125. Their pathology is, however, so obscure, that it will be sufficient to give one or two illustrations of the class of cases to which I refer.

Swan mentions the case of a gentleman who had pains in the backs of his fingers, when evacuating the bladder, if it was much distended. He likewise gives the case of a lady who had pain in the left arm, extending along the course of the ulnar nerve, and apparently dependent on a uterine affection.

Brodie was consulted by a gentleman for severe pain in one instep. On discovering that he also had stricture, and on passing a bougie, the pain in the foot immediately abated, " and in less than a quarter of an hour he left the house free from pain, and walking without the slightest difficulty." This eminent surgeon and his patient are both satisfied that the pain in the foot was connected with the disease of the urethra, and nothing ever relieved it except the introduction of the bougie.

I may briefly notice in this section a class of cases which not very unfrequently, although less commonly than in earlier life, present themselves to the consideration of the physician—I refer to those in which there is an abnormal excitation or diminution of sexual feeling.

An unnatural degree of sexual excitement may exist amongst aged persons of both sexes.

In men it often depends on enlarged prostate or hemorrhoids, and occasionally on the presence of a calculus; it may be much alleviated by proper regimen and medical treatment. In women it is less under medical control, and is frequently associated with disease, or some cause of irritation of the ovaries, uterus, or vagina.* The celebrated Hufeland of Berlin mentions, that he has "seen a very respectable old woman, in her seventieth year, labour under this disease, the cause of which, on dissection, proved to be a scirrhous induration of the ovary." A similar case is given in Bright's *Reports*, and I have reason to believe that in both sexes the disease is more common than is usually supposed. (In reference to this subject I would refer the reader to page 117.)

When the irritation depends on organic disease, we can only hope to alleviate the symptoms. Camphor and hyoscyamus often form a valuable combination in these cases. Acetate of lead is said to be useful, and opium is undoubtedly serviceable. Cold bathing and cold lotions are almost always† useful auxiliaries.

Cases of the opposite character (in the male sex) are of very common occurrence. In a condition of perfect health, the power of which I am speaking continues to the seventieth year, and often considerably later. There are, however, many forms of local and constitutional disease that induce a comparatively premature decay of the energies of the reproductive functions. Some of them will yield to proper treatment; others are irremediable.

I will conclude this Chapter with a few remarks on *uterine hemorrhage in advanced life*. We are often consulted by women considerably past fifty, respecting what they look upon as a return of the monthly courses. This hemorrhage should always be regarded as a serious matter, because, although it often depends on the congested state of the pelvic viscera existing in both sexes in advanced life, it is very frequently connected with organic disease of the uterus. In either case much temporary relief is afforded by strict adherence to

---

* Biett observed a case of this kind in a woman sixty years of age; it depended on prurigo extending to the vagina.

† I should have said "*always useful*," had it not been for the assurance of a lady I recently attended, and in whose statement I can place implicit confidence, that the sensation was always at its height immediately after the use of any local cold application.

the horizontal position, and by slightly elevating the parts affected.* We should ever remember that discharges of every sort must be gently checked in advanced life. The danger resulting from the neglect of this principle is incalculable. A sad illustration of the accuracy of these views occurred recently in my own practice. A lady, aged about seventy, formerly suffered from hemorrhage from the bowels. This was gradually stopped without the least danger. Two years afterwards slight uterine hemorrhage occurred. Her friends became alarmed at what was, in reality, a mere effort of nature for the patient's safety. She was placed under the care of another physician, who checked the hemorrhage, and gave rise to hopeless palsy of the right side of the body.

CHAPTER XII.

SKIN DISEASES, ULCERS, AND SENILE GANGRENE.

SECTION I.

DISEASES OF THE SKIN.

Erythema—Chronic Eczema—Herpes Zoster—Chronic Pemphigus—Rupia—Chronic Ecthyma—Impetigo Sparsa—Acne Rosacea—Prurigo—Psoriasis.

My remarks on this class of diseases will be entirely confined to those forms which have most commonly occurred in my own practice. Skin diseases are most frequent amongst the poor, partly in consequence of the deficient nutrition of the system, and partly in consequence of the comparatively little attention they pay to the condition of the integument; they are, however, by no means confined to persons in any particular class of life.

Erythema is common in advanced life; it is known by the smoothness and tension of the surface, which depend on the œdema of the subcutaneous tissue. It is most frequently seen in the lower extremities, and is sometimes dependent (in women) on varicose veins. It is the *E. læve* of Bateman. I believe it to be simply a modified form

---

* I would refer the reader to an excellent Memoir by M. Gerdy, *On the influence of gravity and a decumbent position on the Circulation, and on Surgical Diseases*, read at the Royal Academy of Medicine, May 25th, 1847.

of œdematous erysipelas. Dropsical limbs, especially when there is abrasion of the cuticle, are frequently affected by it. In aged persons, particularly if they are addicted to intemperate habits, it is liable to pass into ulcers, or even into gangrene.

It is very frequently associated with and, I believe, dependent on a congested state of the abdominal viscera, and till we have duly re-established the secretions and excretions, no treatment will be of much avail. A moderate dose of the *hydrargyrum cum cretâ* with rhubarb, or five grains of Plummer's pill, may be taken at bedtime on alternate nights, and be followed in the morning by a purgative and tonic draught.* Two or three doses of a mild mercurial, such as I have indicated, are usually sufficient in the first instance; it is, however, often necessary to recur to this treatment at intervals, if the liver presents signs of torpidity. The vegetable tonics may then be prescribed, either alone or in combination with chlorate of potash, the preparations of ammonia, &c. A nourishing diet and wine must be allowed. With regard to local applications, it is difficult to lay down any general rules. Warm stimulating embrocations are most commonly useful; but I have seen many cases where they caused irritation, and in which nothing gave so much relief as the *liquor plumbi diacetatis dilutus*, applied lukewarm. It is essential to the success of the treatment that the limb should be retained in a horizontal or slightly elevated position.

Chronic Eczema is an affection I have occasionally seen in persons of advanced life. A woman, aged sixty-seven, of broken-down constitution, and with the eruption marked on all the extremities, was under my care during the early part of the present year (1848). She had been suffering from it for a year and a half, and tried numerous remedies. There was extreme itching, and on some spots an abundant exudation of ichorous discharge. The whole appearance of the woman was cachectic; the tongue was foul, the bowels costive, and the urine loaded with urate of ammonia. The disease completely disappeared in less than a month under the external application of weak tar ointment,† and the daily administration of the infusion and com-

---

* Combinations of the infusion of gentian, or of the various preparations of bark, with the compound infusion of senna, answer excellently in these cases. I am likewise in the habit of regulating the bowels after the more active treatment described in the text, with the confection of senna, to which I add sulphur and powdered bark.

† I began with ℨij. of the *unguentum picis* to an ounce of lard, and increased it till they were used in equal proportions.

pound tincture of bark, with a sufficient quantity of the compound infusion of senna to keep the bowels properly open. She complained afterwards of slight headaches, which were removed by the occasional application of a small blister (kept open for a few days) to the back of the neck.

This disease is not unfrequently seen behind the ears, and, in women, on the perineum.

Herpes Zoster is a disease of which I generally see three or four cases annually in old persons. These cases almost invariably occur in the summer or early autumn. This affection is now more troublesome than in earlier life. The constitutional disturbance preceding the eruption is often severe, and the vesicles assume a larger form, and the sores left by them are not easy to heal. The general treatment must be the same as for the preceding skin-diseases. When the heat and stinging are very severe, a lotion containing opium gives great relief. If there is a tendency to ulceration, nitrate of silver should be applied locally. Neuralgic pains are often felt for months in the seat of the eruption.

Herpes Preputialis is not uncommon, especially in cases of irritability of the bladder.

Chronic Pemphigus affects chiefly persons advanced in age and of debilitated constitution. The eruption is preceded for a few days by a feeling of discomfort and sickness, and by pains in the head, back, and limbs. There is also disturbance of the bowels, and not unfrequently we observe either pain and difficulty in micturition, or bloody urine.

The eruption appears at first in the form of small red spots, accompanied by some itching; the cuticle at these spots soon becomes elevated, and a bulla as large as a nut, and often much larger, is soon formed. These bullæ contain a pale yellowish serous fluid, which if not discharged by their bursting, becomes reddish on the third or fourth day, while the bullæ themselves shrivel up. In the latter case there is a dark scab, while in the former there is a sore and excoriated surface. These bullæ continue to rise either on different parts of the body in succession, or on the same part for several weeks, so that they may commonly be seen in every stage of development.

This disease is sometimes complicated with herpes and prurigo; in the latter case it is a most distressing affection, from the intense itching which accompanies the eruption.

It has been observed by Erasmus Wilson, and I fully concur with him in the remark, that this eruption is an effort of the system to rid itself of some morbid disposition. I have seen it in one patient twice precede an attack of low gout; and there can, I think, be no doubt, that it is always dependent on an impure condition of the circulating fluids.

The constitutional treatment must depend upon the causes, as far as we can ascertain them, that are exerting a noxious influence on the circulating fluids. Wine, bark, with or without sulphuric acid, and light nutritious animal food are imperatively called for, when the disease occurs in aged, worn-out patients.

The topical treatment consists in puncturing the bullæ in an early stage, and applying warm fomentations. The surface may then be treated by an absorbent powder, or a mildly astringent lotion. Warm baths—either simple or alkaline—are usually of much service. When the irritation is very distressing, anodynes must be freely used externally and internally.

Rupia escharotica occasionally develops itself in advanced life. The preceding remarks on the causes and treatment of chronic pemphigus are equally applicable to this affection.

Chronic Ecthyma and *Impetigo sparsa*, are affections depending on the same class of depressing causes, and to be treated in the same manner as the two preceding diseases. In *Impetigo* the crusts sometimes attain a great thickness, and quite encase the affected part. Dr. Copland has very judiciously recalled the attention of the profession to the internal use of tar-water in these and other chronic skin-diseases.

I now come to the consideration of a disease that is comparatively frequent in the middle and advanced periods of life, and that from the disfigurement it causes, is very annoying to the patient; I refer to *Acne rosacea*, popularly known as *carbuncled face*, *rosy drop*, &c. It is confined almost exclusively to the face, and usually to the nose, and parts of the cheeks adjoining it. It seldom occurs before the meridian of life, and is often seen in females at the critical period. In persons predisposed to this affection the point of the nose is first observed to become unusually red after meals, or after any stimulus or excitement. The redness by degrees becomes habitual, and is most marked towards evening. The skin gradually thickens, the veins of the nose enlarge, and the surface is uneven and granulated. There is more or less finely comminuted desquamation going on, and small indurations and yellow pustules are scattered over the reddened surface. The nose becomes much enlarged and of a fiery red, and subsequently of a livid colour. The nostrils are distended, and the alæ fissured or divided into several separate lobes. In very old people the nodular indurations often become the seat of intractable ulcerations.

The prognosis of this affection is, on the whole, unfavourable.

It is impossible, in many cases, to distinguish the cause of *Acne rosacea*. While it may often be traced to an undue enjoyment of the pleasures of the table, to habits of intemperance, to the suppression of some habitual discharge, or to the influence of certain modes of life requiring much exposure to heat, cases sometimes present themselves in which it cannot be referred to any of these causes, and where, moreover, there is no hereditary tendency towards it.

With regard to treatment, I may observe that more depends on the diet and general regimen than on medicine. We should strongly urge the adoption of a mild farinaceous diet, with a small portion of easily digestible animal food, while the beverage should consist of toast and water, or barley-water. Tea, coffee, beer, wine, and spirits must be strictly interdicted. Gentle and regular exercise, and due attention to the condition of the skin and abdominal viscera, are also essentially requisite for the removal of this affection.

The French dermatologists have recommended the application of very weak lotions or baths of nitro-muriatic acid. Stimulants are sure to be productive of harm ; and, perhaps, the vapour-douche is the best as well as the safest local application.

Prurigo is the next affection to be noticed. I have already referred to this disease, or at least to certain varieties of it, in pages 143 and 175. It is an affection easily recognised by the distinct papulæ differing scarcely in colour from the skin, and accompanied with sharp, burning itching, of the most intolerable kind. It generally occurs about the shoulders, back, and neck, but sometimes the whole cutaneous surface is attacked. When the extremities are affected, the disease is generally very severe. Dermatologists have distinguished three varieties, *Prurigo mitis*, *P. formicans*, and *P. senilis*. The two former differ merely in degree, while the third presents certain peculiarities. The following remarks apply to the two first forms. The itching which is continually felt becomes aggravated towards evening, and especially by the warmth of bed : it has been compared to that which might be produced by innumerable ants gnawing the skin; hence the name *formicans*. The patients, in trying to find relief, tear the papulæ with their nails, and a minute drop of blood oozes out, forming a thin black scab. In old persons prurigo often continues for two or three years, or even longer. It gradually spreads over the greater part of the body, and the papulæ are large, hard, prominent, and blackish from the effused blood.

The eruption is accompanied with considerable thickening of the skin, and is attended with occasional exacerbations, during which the papulæ often become confluent. The skin becomes inflamed, vesicles, pustules, and boils are often developed ; and abscesses are even occasionally formed.

This is the kind of prurigo most commonly met with in aged persons, and which I am always in the habit of regarding as *Prurigo senilis;* but Biett, Cazenave, and other French writers restrict this term to a form in which the papulæ scarcely differ from those I have described ; they add, however, that " the dryness of the skin, which is mere accidental in *P. formicans*, is a specific character of *P. senilis;* but the leading distinction is the swarm of insects with which the skin is infested in the latter affection."

The causes of prurigo are much the same as those of the preceding skin-disease—bad nourishment, want of cleanliness, impurity of the blood. I need not revert to the constitutional treatment required in these cases, further than to remind the reader that this affection is often accompanied (if not preceded) by a diminished secretion of urine, and that this circumstance may furnish us with a hint in reference to treatment. In addition to regulating the biliary secretion, we must try the effects of diuretics. (See page 177.) A great deal may sometimes be effected by the use of the alkaline salts with a decoction of juniper berries or broom, by squills, or by more powerful stimulants, as turpentine or cantharides. To improve the general tone of the system we may give the decoction of sarsaparilla and nitric acid, and allow a mild nutritious diet. All heating food and stimulating drinks must be avoided.

With regard to external applications I can lay down no general rules. A lather of soap and hot water rubbed over the affected parts with a sponge or soft brush night and morning is often productive of much comfort. Dr. Graves recommends that we should subsequently have recourse to a lotion composed of a pint of whiskey and a drachm of laudanum, to be applied hot, with a sponge, at bedtime. Dr. Bellingham has recently advised the local application of creosote,

---

* *Manual of Diseases of the Skin*, by Cazenave and Schedel, translated by Burgess, p. 195.

either as an ointment, consisting of ten, or from that to twenty minims, with an ounce of lard; or as a lotion, consisting of twenty or thirty minims, with an ounce of spirit of wine and nine ounces of water. Lotions and ointments, containing the alkaline carbonates, iodide of potassium, muriate of ammonia, bichloride of mercury, hydrocyanic acid, preparations of opium, &c. &c. have been at different times recommended, and are undoubtedly deserving of trial. The use of the warm bath should never be neglected.

In those cases where pediculi or other insects are observed, sulphur baths must be freely used.

Lichen agrius is occasionally observed in persons advanced in life. The treatment I have just described is here equally applicable. In many cases of skin disease, in which itching is a troublesome symptom, considerable relief is often afforded by the lotion recommended by Dr. Graves, of eight ounces of decoction of poppies and two or three drachms of solution of isinglass.

Psoriasis is the last skin-disease requiring notice. It is an affection I commonly meet with in the declining years of life, and that is often associated with the gouty diathesis; and I can by no means subscribe to the accuracy of the statement of Cazenave, " that it is very rare to see a squamous eruption first show itself after the age of fifty."*

Psoriasis, when extensive, is usually preceded by the ordinary symptoms of constitutional disorder, and requires the same general treatment as the preceding diseases. There are very few cases that will not yield to arsenic, but as this is a medicine which is not so well borne in advanced life as in adult age, I always try other means previously. Pitch, a very old remedy for the squamous diseases, has been successful in two cases in which I have tried it, but has failed in others. It may be given in pills with liquorice powder, or in capsules. The prolonged and free use of tar-water will probably yield the same result. Liquor potassæ, iodide of potassium, bichloride of mercury, tincture of cantharides, &c., have been found useful by different practitioners. Cod-liver oil, if the stomach will bear it, is often highly serviceable. When all other remedies seem inert, and we are obliged to have recourse to arsenic, we may commence with three minims of Fowler's solution, taken after meals, in two ounces of decoction of dulcamara. The dose must be gradually

---

* *Ann. des Mal. de la Peau.* tom. 1. p. 133. Paris, 1844.

increased till irritation of the eyes, heat in the region of the stomach, &c., show that the arsenic is acting on the system. The medicine must then be suspended till these symptoms subside. An aggravation of the eruption frequently precedes a cure.

When the above treatment fails, we may try arsenic in the solid form of pill—the Asiatic pill; and finally Donovan's *Liquor Arsenici et Hydrargyri Iodidi.*

Blisters applied over the patches often improve the condition of the skin. A case lately occurred in my hands in which a large circular patch on the nates of a woman aged fifty-nine, who had taken cod-liver oil for three weeks, did not improve in appearance till the thermic treatment was several times applied to the apparently healthy surrounding skin. I have lately used a lotion of glycerine, as recommended by Mr. Startin, with considerable advantage. If one great use of local applications be to protect the parts from the action of the air, collodion will probably be found serviceable. Hot water, vapour or sulphur baths are always an important auxiliary to the treatment of these and all other chronic skin-diseases.

In the squamous diseases attention to diet is of the greatest importance.

SECTION II.

On Ulcers of the Legs.

I HAVE so frequently alluded to the danger resulting in many cases from the healing of ulcers and other discharging surfaces, in persons of advanced life, that any remarks on the cure of this class of affections might almost seem out of place in this volume. In reviewing the works that have been devoted to this subject by Whately, Baynton, Home, and others, it cannot however fail to strike us that in many cases ulcers in very aged persons were cured, and those persons lived for many years afterwards enjoying an improved state of health. "I have ventured," says Dr. Underwood, "to cure ulcers of many years' standing in very old people, and one, many years ago, in a lady upwards of eighty years of age, whom a very eminent surgeon had cautioned against suffering it to be healed; all of whom have since enjoyed good health, and the ulcers have shown no disposition to break out again." The point for the physician to decide is simply this—Is the ulcer a natural issue, and intended as a safeguard to the system? Or is it a consequence of debility, languid circulation, &c.? In the latter case, he can be doing little harm to the constitution in attempting a cure, provided that he pays especial attention to the general health for some time subsequently, and at once establishes an issue, if he observes any tendency to cerebral congestion. Tepid water-dressing, and due support by bandaging, constitute the requisite treatment. When the ulcers are very irritable, opium may be freely administered.

SECTION III.

Senile Gangrene.

THIS disease usually occurs in those parts which are most remote from the heart, and in which, therefore, the circulation most readily flags. It is most commonly observed to commence on the toes, more rarely on the fingers, and, occasionally, but very seldom, on the nose or organs of generation.

There are certain premonitory symptoms, which are of a purely local character. The patient first complains of severe and continuous pain, depriving him of sleep; this pain is sometimes confined to the toe, and is sometimes felt over the whole foot; and it is frequently preceded or accompanied by a feeling of dulness, pricking, and want of sensation in the part. No pulse can be felt in the affected limb which feels cold to the patient; and its temperature is actually diminished, in consequence of the impeded circulation that always exists in these cases. The foot sometimes assumes a livid tint before the commencement of gangrene.

There is now usually formed on one of the small toes a dark-coloured vesicle, which is accompanied with considerable pain, and soon bursts, exposing a dark, livid, slightly moist surface. This surface extends, other vesicles spring up, and large portions of epidermis are thrown off. This, however, is not invariably the case. Sometimes the affected part assumes a shrivelled, mummified appearance, and no vesicles are produced; it is cold and dead, and on cutting it little or no blood escapes. This dry form is most common in the poorer and ill-fed classes, whilst in those who are in a comfortable position in life, the former or moist form predominates.

In both forms the adjacent parts are œdematous, more or less livid, and cold; in the moist, the pain is by far the more severe, and febrile symptoms are more commonly present. There is always great prostration of strength, a small and feeble pulse, a dry, blackish tongue, a sensation of internal cold, which nothing can remove, and a peculiar fœtor about the excretions.

Such are the characters of the premonitory symptoms, and of the disease itself; but if the disease has not by this time produced a fatal result, a third state—that of reaction—is established. An inflamed border is formed round the mortified part, and in the moist form the gangrenous portion becomes soft and putrid, while in the dry form it becomes more or less detached.

Senile gangrene, as we most commonly see it, is a mixture of these two forms.

We occasionally meet with some difficulty in diagnosing this affection at an early stage, in consequence of the limb sometimes being perfectly paralysed for some days before the appearance of any physical signs. The following considerations will however enable us to distinguish between this and nervous paralysis. The paralysis of sensation and motion from the suspension of the arterial circulation is complete; while the paralysis dependent on lesions of the nerves or nervous centres, is usually more or less incomplete. Moreover, the peculiar coldness of the part, and the circumstance that there is no arterial pulsation, and that the vessel feels like a piece of string, aid us in our diagnosis.

Erysipelas can hardly be taken for senile gangrene. The parts it affects (see page 187) are different, and its ravages do not extend to tissues deeper than the skin.

Any cause that impedes the free access of arterial blood may give rise to this disease, as petrifaction (falsely called ossification) or local coarctation of the larger arterial stems, diminution and obliteration of the smaller vessels, stoppage of the arteries by fibrinous coagula, any impediment to the return of the blood through the veins, diminution of the heart's power (fatty or atrophied heart, &c.); in short, the affection seems to depend on the separation and deposition of fibrin obstructing the circulation. There is no subject on which there exists a greater difference of opinion than regarding the treatment of senile gangrene. While the French pathologists look upon the disease as inflammatory, and treat it by scarification, leeching, venesection, and other antiphlogistic measures, it has until recently been the habit in this country to allow a full nutritious diet, and the free use of stimulants.

The line of treatment in which I feel the greatest confidence is very much the same as that advocated by Professor Syme. In order to arrest the morbid action (which seems to be a combination of weakness and over-action to the affected part), it is necessary to lower the tendency to excitement throughout the system, by enforcing a strictly vegetable and milk diet, abstinence from every sort of stimulant, the free use of opiates as long as the pain continues, the maintenance of perfect quiet in the horizontal or in a slightly elevated position, and the application of a poultice or of a thick covering of cotton or wool to the affected part.

The following case occurred in the clinical wards of the Edinburgh Infirmary during the period I was studying in that city, and was subsequently published by Professor Syme. I give it in a condensed form, as illustrating the line of practice above referred to.

Helen Byres, a very thin, weak old woman, stating her age to be fifty-seven, but apparently much older, was admitted on the 28th of January. She complained of severe pain in her left foot, especially in the little and great toes. The instep was red, and somewhat swelled, and extremely tender to pressure. The little toe was quite black, and the great one of a dark purplish colour. The former had become painful two or three weeks previously, and after eight days of continued and increasing pain, discoloration was first noticed; it was only a few days previous to admission that she had been suddenly seized with violent pain in the ball of the great toe. During the first week of her residence in the Infirmary she was treated by the surgeon's clerk with nourishing food and wine; but the pain, redness, and swelling of the foot increased, and the dark discoloration of the toes became more extensive. It was not till this time that Mr. Syme's attention was directed to the case. "Having ascertained," he observes, "the nature of the complaint, I did not hesitate to order a strictly farinaceous diet, water for drink, and a simple poultice for the foot. The symptoms then gradually abated, and the patient, instead of sinking under the united effect of disease and weakness, as she had previously threatened to do, acquired additional strength, and greatly improved in her appearance. In the beginning of March the little toe separated at its metatarsal joint, and about three months afterwards the great toe did the same. The sores healed kindly, and presented on each side of the foot a no less seemly cicatrix than if a skilful amputation had been performed. The starving plan was then abandoned; and the poor old woman, after subsisting on bread and water for upwards of four months, was allowed the usual diet of the hospital."

Further experience has confirmed the advantages of this course of treatment, notwithstanding the opposition it has met with at the hands of some of the metropolitan surgeons;* and I full concur in the observation of Mr. Syme, that " the advantage almost immediately derived from abandoning the use of animal food, with its stimulating accompaniments of wine and spirits, is so obvious, that this plan of treatment requires only a commencement to insure its continuance."

I have often met with cases in which there have been certain premonitory symptoms of senile gangrene—a slight blueness in the toes or fingers, pain on motion or pressure, and rigidity of the arteries. In these cases mild tonics and a moderate proportion of animal food are undoubtedly serviceable, and prevent the accession of the disease. I have at the present time a poor woman, aged seventy-nine, under my care, who for nearly three years has had this tendency.

CHAPTER XIII.

ON GOUT AND RHEUMATISM.

As *acute gout* usually makes its first attack during the prime of life, I shall not treat of it as a disease generally, but only touch upon those peculiarities which it presents in advanced years. With respect to the nature of the disease I may premise that we have undoubted evidence of the existence of a *materies morbi* (most probably uric acid or urate of soda, combined with other organic matter), capable of accumulation in the system, of change of place within the body, and of removal from it.†

When acute gout first shows itself in advanced life, it is more commonly acquired than hereditary, and is usually not so amenable to

---

* In the recent well-known trial of Baker *v.* Lowe, the treatment advocated in the text was, however, supported by Liston, Lawrence, Aston Key, Skey, &c.

† See Holland's *Notes and Reflections*, 2d Ed. p. 124. Dr. Garrod has recently succeeded in separating the crystals of uric acid from the blood in these cases.

treatment as at an earlier period. From my own experience I should say, that when the primary attack occurs in advanced life, the premonitory symptoms continue for a longer period than ordinary, and that the paroxysm is more acute. The treatment is often strangely empirical in these cases. A patient will recount a series of symptoms resembling those premonitory of gout, and which would be perfectly explicable if he had suffered from that disease, or even if it existed in his family; the physician too often prescribes merely for the symptoms, but in this he is not to blame, for he has no clue to the real origin of the disease, and only adopts a course that in many of the affections of old age is the wisest.

The most common of these symptoms are flatulence, oppression after a meal, and a very irregular appetite, varying from voracity to anorexia; heart-burn, with the acidity of the stomach, and acid eructations; the spirits are usually depressed; there is drowsiness during the day, and during the night the sleep is broken and unrefreshing; the bowels are generally costive, and the urine scanty and high-coloured.

These symptoms may (especially in first attacks) last only for a day or two, or indeed be hardly noticed; but they more frequently extend for weeks, or even months, and their import remains misunderstood till their sudden disappearance on the occurrence of an attack of gout in the extremities at length reveals their true nature.

During the fit the bowels are generally confined, and the stools, which are rather of a pale or dark green colour, are extremely offensive; micturition is often painful, and the urine scanty, high-coloured, and very acid, depositing an abundant sediment of urates. As the œdema and redness subside, the cuticle of the affected part desquamates—a process which is often attended with very annoying itching.

This disorder, as is well known, is almost sure to return. There is generally an interval of at least a year or two, and occasionally of a much longer period between the first three or four attacks, but these intervals gradually shorten; the attacks become annual (often occurring with singular regularity), semestral, and, finally, more protracted as they are more frequent; they leave the patient scarcely free from the disease except for a month or two in the summer.

I shall say nothing of the predisposing causes of gout. They have been fully developed by innumerable writers, and I could offer nothing new upon the subject. A slight reference to some of the most important will be found in my subsequent remarks on the mode of treatment to be pursued during the intervals of comparative health. The exciting causes must, however, be noticed, since by knowing them the patient may possibly avoid them. A paroxysm will often immediately follow upon any excessive indulgence at table. I have frequently had patients who are fully aware of the certain consequences that would ensue from their drinking two or three glasses of champagne. A gentleman, aged about sixty, who is frequently under my care, almost invariably finds that in cold weather a single glass will produce a weakness and a twitching pain in one of his ankles; he has never had an attack of gout, which, however, exists in his family, but frequently suffers from slight asthmatic attacks, which succeed any deviation from his ordinary regular mode of living, and yield more readily to minute doses of colchicum, combined with blue pill, than to any other remedy. For a gouty person, champagne is the very worst wine that can be taken, and next to it, claret. The free and regular use of ale or porter at meal times, and port wine after dinner, will excite it in persons of the gouty disposition unless regular active exercise by taken. It may be observed that malt liquors and wine are not only injurious in themselves, but also in a secondary manner, by stimulating the stomach, and thus leading to excess in relation to food as well as to drink, to an extent almost equally prejudicial. Mental or bodily fatigue, or both combined, often induce a paroxysm. It is well known that Sydenham's exertions in writing his tract on gout brought on an attack of the disease. Powerful mental emotions, whether exciting or depressing, may bring it on, while they may also, as we shall presently see, cause the disease to assume an irregular form after it has been established. I could mention several cases that have fallen under my own observation, in which bodily fatigue has been the exciting cause; thus gout in persons addicted to field-sports often regularly comes on with the commencement of the hunting or shooting season. Any circumstance tending to check the due action of the excreting organs may bring it on. Gout has been often known to follow constipation of the bowels, checked perspiration, and the sudden suppression of bleeding piles. The last exciting cause to which I shall refer is external injury. The first attack is often at the seat of an old sprain or bruise; and Dr. Heberden even goes so far as to say that he believes he has actually seen an attack of gout brought on by the bite of a flea.

The only diseases for which acute gout can be mistaken, are acute rheumatism, which is very rare in advanced life, and, possibly, common inflammation of the joints. An experienced practitioner can, however, hardly fall into error on this point.

The treatment may be considered under three heads: (1) that of the premonitory symptoms, (2) that of the paroxysm, and (3), that after the paroxysm, with the view of preventing a recurrence of the attack.

I believe that, for some time previous to an attack, the liver is generally torpid and congested, that there are accumulated fæces in the large intestines, that the digestive mucous membrane is in an irritable condition, and that the blood is loaded with effete matter. Most authors recommend venesection in such cases; there may be cases in which it is advisable, but in most instances a few leeches applied to the anus, will produce at least equally good effects, without depressing the patient. If the patient have suffered from a hemorrhoidal discharge, we should attempt to re-establish it by aloetic purgatives; and where these fail, aloetic injections sometimes succeed. If the tongue be very foul, and the patient suffer from heart-burn, a mild emetic (fifteen grains of ipecacuanha) is frequently useful, where there is no pain or tenderness in the epigastric region, and if none of the causes which often render the action of emetics dangerous to old persons, as hernia, for instance, be present. Purgatives are always of service in these cases, although the patient may declare that the bowels are regularly open. I usually prescribe a combination of calomel and blue pill (two or three grains of each) to be taken at bedtime, and a warm stomachic purgative the following morning. By the occasional repetition of these means, together with moderate diet, regular exercise, and care in guarding against mental or bodily fatigue, a threatened attack may be often averted, and always mitigated.

With respect to the treatment during the paroxysm, it must be recollected that I am speaking of gout as it occurs in advanced life. I shall say nothing of blood-letting, further than that even in adult life, and in strong constitutions, I have never seen any decided benefit from it. Although leeches applied to the affected joint mitigate the pain, they also prolong the attack. Neither shall I notice the innumerable medicines—the purgatives, emetics, diuretics, diaphoretics, and narcotics—that have at different times been recommended in the treatment of this disease. I will simply give the course of treatment which experience has shown to be most commonly efficacious. The three great points to be attended to, are to regulate the action of the liver and bowels by mild mercurials and warm aromatic purgatives, to relieve pain by means of opiates, or in very severe cases, when the patient's tortures prevent sleep, by chloroform, and to diminish the local inflammation by colchicum.

In prescribing colchicum for aged persons, there are two points which must not be disregarded. Frequent previous use may enable patients in advanced life to bear with advantage larger doses even than adults unaccustomed to it; and conversely a very small dose (especially if not associated with a carminative) may produce extreme prostration. Ought colchicum to be administered at the commencement of the attack? We have high authorities on both sides of the question. In old persons, especially when there is much derangement of the liver and bowels, it is safer to relieve those organs before we administer colchicum. When this has been satisfactorily accomplished, we may order fifteen minims or a scruple of the wine of the cormus (Vin. Colch. Ph. L.) to be taken twice a-day with a little magnesia in any appropriate vehicle; and at bed-time, if there is no apparent depression nor irritability of the bowels, two or three grains of the acetous extract with compound extract of colocynth and calomel, or with Dover's powder, as the case may seem to require. In persons of irritable habits, broken constitution, and advanced age, the nocturnal pain must be soothed; and if for any reason opium should be contra-indicated, the extract of Indian hemp, or a brief inhalation of chloroform may be substituted for it. The purgative should in most cases be repeated twice or thrice in the week, and may either consist of a few grains of calomel and blue pill at night, and a warm aperient in the morning, or if the patient be strong enough to bear it, two or three grains of calomel may be made into a couple of pills with an equal quantity of resin of scammony, and four or five grains of the compound extract of colocynth. The colchicum must be continued in the above manner till the termination of the attack (provided it excite neither vomiting, purging, nor great prostration), and for some time afterwards in smaller quantity.

Various modifications of treatment will suggest themselves to the experienced practitioner; thus, if there is much febrile disturbance present, it must be met by small doses of tartar emetic, sweet spirits of nitre, or spirit of Mindererus, which may either be given alone, or with colchicum. Again we often meet with instances in which colchicum can only be borne when combined with an opiate; in these cases the bowels require especial attention.

Dr. Seymour has recently recalled the attention of the profession to the use of the Decoction of Burdock root (Arctium Minus Ph. D.) " as an adjunct to other remedies, and in acute gout." The following are his directions on the subject. Two ounces of the sliced root are well washed, and are *slowly* boiled in a pint and a half of water; the fluid is reduced to a pint, and then strained. This pint is to be drank in the course of the twenty-four hours. If the patient does not object to the increased quantity of the fluid, it may be mixed with an equal bulk of milk. It should be continued for several weeks.

My remarks would be incomplete were I to omit all notice of local applications. When the tension of the skin is very great, I usually recommend that the part should be kept moist with sweet or castor oil. I do not know, however, that the latter is any better than the former. I have likewise found that relief is sometimes afforded from the application of combed wool, and swansdown; in like manner the pain is often very considerably mitigated by rolling the affected part in oil-silk; but in old persons with a dry skin, it sometimes rather increases than diminishes suffering. There is a large mass of evidence in favour of the application of the moxa during the paroxysm, but I have no personal experience of its effects in these cases. I have frequently prescribed small blisters about the size of a crown piece to the joint with very obvious advantage, at the commencement of the fit. The local abstraction of the serum often gives considerable relief. Although putting the foot in cold water, and the applying refrigerant lotions may undoubtedly allay the intensity of the pain, it is to be feared that this fool-hardy practice has too frequently resulted in apoplexy, paralysis, and gout in the vital organs.

The diet, during the paroxysm, must be very much regulated by the condition of the patient. Arrow-root and sago, combined in many cases with a little sherry, or even brandy, are sufficient for the first two or three days of the fit; broth and light puddings may then be generally allowed, while the use of wine must be in a considerable degree influenced by the ordinary habits of the patient. A wish to exchange the bed for the sofa or easy chair is almost always to be encouraged, for there is usually more harm done by remaining in bed too long than too short a time. The first exercise of the limb should be very gentle. It may be remarked that when the patient complains of the pressure of the bed-clothes, a cradle should always be procured.

We have still to notice the treatment during convalescence, and, if the attacks are common, in the intervals between them. This consists for the most part, in the proper management and regulation of the digestive organs. The decoction of burdock may (according to Dr. Seymour) be taken with advantage* for weeks, and ten or fifteen minims of wine of colchicum given at bed-time.

If the affected part still exhibits swelling and weakness, it should be sponged night and morning with a lukewarm and strong solution of salt in water, and after being wiped dry, should be rubbed with the hand for some time, and then enveloped in a bandage. When the immediate effects of the fit are over, we find the stomach weak and unable to discharge its ordinary functions. This is the stage at which, from time immemorial, bitters have been recommended. I need not revert to the Portland powder, and to the similar compounds that have at various periods found favour with the public. Dr. Seymour states, that "where a very excellent stomachic bitter is required, when attacks of gout have left a weak state of the stomach, the infusion of the *menyanthes trifoliata* has been found to restore the languid digestion and broken strength."

From my own experience of its value in the many cases in which I have tried it, and of its great utility in certain allied morbid conditions, I can speak highly of sulphur, half a drachm of which should be taken regularly twice a-day in a little milk, as recommended by Cheyne. Its good effects more than counterbalance any little unpleasantness it may cause the patient. While taking this medicine, all chills should be avoided and warm clothing adhered to. The same precautions are requisite while taking compound medicines in which sulphur is a leading ingredient. There is a well-known empirical remedy, whose action, it would appear from the formula given by Dr. Paris, is chiefly owing to this substance. I refer to "the Chelsea Pensioner."† It is composed of Guaiacum Resin, ʒi., Powdered Rhubarb, ʒij., Cream of Tartar, ʒi., Flowers of Sulphur, ʒi.; one Nutmeg finely powdered; made into an electuary with one pound of clarified honey: two large spoonfuls to be taken night and morning.

* I believe that in many cases (for instance in gout, chronic skin-diseases, &c.) we might produce a much more marked effect on the system by adhering to the plan adopted a century or two ago, of administering infusions and decoctions by the pint or even by the quart, than by prescribing what are presumed to be equivalents of extracts, active principles, &c., in a concentrated form.

† It is said to be the prescription of a Chelsea Pensioner, by which Lord Amherst was cured. Dr. Seymour, on the authority of Mr. Keate, gives a somewhat different formula.

The daily use of rhubarb with alkalies and a tonic* is commonly very serviceable.

There is one common error against which I have frequently had occasion to warn my gouty patients. It is with reference to their diet. While in many cases a fit of gout is excited by the too free use of animal food, the practitioner must never forget that it may be produced by too low a system of living. Amongst the poorer classes I have often found nothing so serviceable in keeping off the gout as a little animal food and a glass of porter daily. I have ascertained that the first attack has frequently been contemporaneous with the period of their getting out of work, and being in a more destitute state than usual, and I have seen such patients at once improve (even if the fit be at its height) from the time they have received due nourishment. Now this affords us a useful lesson. It shows that we may over-starve our patients, and that in attempting too strenuously to keep the enemy at bay, we may be only weakening our own defences. Hence, when consulted by a patient on this subject, we must warn him against excesses in either direction; and further, we must lay fully as much stress on the importance of attention to the *quantity* as to the *quality* of his food.

In addition to a due attention to diet, every one who has suffered from gout should take especial care that the liver, bowels, kidneys, and skin properly discharge their functions. But I have so frequently had occasion to advert to these points and to the means of regulating these functions, that I need say nothing further in this place regarding them.

Chronic gout, although occasionally a primary affection, is usually a consequence of previous acute attacks, either when they have not terminated in the ordinary paroxysm, or when the constitution has been much enfeebled from the effect of repeated seizures. In this form of gout the colour of the affected part is little altered, sometimes not at all. The pains in the joints, for more than one is often affected, is less acute and more wandering than in the preceding form, and often alternates with pain and cramp in the stomach. In most respects the symptoms are analogous to, but much less intense than those of acute gout. The general health is usually more disturbed. It is this form of gout which most commonly leads to the formation of

* The following is a formula I often employ in these cases :—℞. Pulv. Rhei., gr. vi. Sodæ Carb. gr. xv. Pulv. Calumbæ, gr. iv. M. Fiat. pulvis ante prand. sumend.

concretions (chalkstones as they are commonly called) around the joints.

The treatment must be conducted on much the same principles as in acute gout: the secretions must be properly regulated; colchicum should be given in less frequent and in smaller doses; and diuretics* often appear to be of signal service. When the more urgent symptoms are removed, sulphur either alone or with guaiacum, and iodide of potassium with *liquor potassæ* in the compound decoction of sarsaparilla, are amongst our most valuable remedies. Direct tonics, as for instance the milder preparations of iron, may often be given with great service, when the secretions have been properly regulated.

Local applications are of more value in chronic than in acute gout. Stimulating liniments may be rubbed in with much advantage in cases of an indolent nature: galvanism is reported to have been found useful, and I have frequently seen the good effects of painting the affected part with an alcoholic solution of iodine, which must, however, be considerably stronger than that of the London Pharmacopœia. Galvanism and iodine are, however, only of service after the local pain has nearly subsided.

The concretions that are frequently deposited after numerous attacks of chronic gout often defy all the resources of our art. I have seen more advantage from the prolonged application of nitrate of silver to the joint, together with an occasional leech, and the frequent immersion of the part in hot water (a quarter of an hour morning and night) than from any other means.

Irregular gout, the most important of the three varieties, now claims our attention. It may be conveniently arranged under two heads: the first including cases in which certain symptoms are relieved by the occurrence of a paroxysm of gout; and the second, the derangements consequent upon a sudden, entire or partial cessation of the paroxysm.

In reference to the first head, I may remark that cases abound in the various treatises on this disease, and in a more or less marked degree must have occurred to all who have had any experience in practice, in which affections, often of the most dangerous character, have at once disappeared on the occurrence of a regular attack of gout.

Severe cases of palpitation of the heart (of course not dependent

---

* Benzoic acid either alone or neutralised with ammonia is an admirable diuretic in these cases.

on structural diseases of that organ) that have defied all the ordinary modes of treatment, very often disappear spontaneously on an access of genuine gout. Various affections of the kidney and bladder, asthma, prolonged symptoms of the most distressing dyspepsia, hypochondriasis, and occasionally head-symptoms of the most alarming nature, have also, as if by magic retired, on the supervention of a paroxysm of gout. I quote the following lines from Dr. Seymour's remarks on gout, as they very clearly describe the nature of these cases. " Rarely in *acquired* gout, often in hereditary, the following occurs : a patient suffers from most acute and constant pain in the stomach, he has great loss of appetite, and the taking of food is followed by torture ; after a time gout appears in the extremities, and he is immediately freed from his distress ! Another is exposed suddenly, feeling well, to blasts of cold air : his throat becomes swollen and *extremely painful*, deglutition is almost impossible ; there is fever, *extreme depression*, almost despair ; no local cause can be discovered sufficient for the severity of the symptoms. Suddenly great relief is afforded to the pain in the throat, swallowing becomes easy, and gout appears in the foot or hand." In other cases there may be no local pain, but at the same time, the most alarming symptoms, as for instance, very violent and frightful attacks of hiccough continuing for several days, or constant vomiting with coldness of the extremities and a pulse too rapid to be counted (Seymour). Dr. Copland relates the following interesting case, bearing forcibly on this point. He was called to see a gentleman who was seized in the evening with symptoms of complete congestive apoplexy, for which he was bled and purged, but without restoration to his consciousness. On the following morning gout suddenly appeared for the first time with great intensity in the ball of the great toe of the right foot, and instantly removed all the apoplectic symptoms, the mental faculties becoming perfectly clear and undisturbed.

No general rules can be laid down for the treatment of such cases, further than that if from past experience we know the patient to be of a gouty habit, we must use our best endeavours by warm foot-baths, rubefacients, &c. to establish gout in the feet. Colchicum is seldom admissible.

Under the second head we have to consider the derangements consequent upon a sudden, entire or partial cessation of the paroxysm. This is *retrocedent gout*. In these cases the stomach and intestines are the organs by far the most commonly attacked. The lungs, kidneys, bladder, and head are more rarely affected.

In treating these cases there are two points to be borne in mind: (1) if possible, to recall the gout to the extremity from which it has migrated, and (2) to apply suitable remedies to allay the pain in the organ secondarily attacked. When the stomach is affected, opium in large doses may be given; and the frequent vomiting that occurs in these cases is best met by effervescing draughts, to which, if necessary, two or three minims of hydrocyanic acid may be added. The collapse attendant on these cases is most successfully combated by the free use of hot brandy and water. Occasionally ammonia must be resorted to. There is at times a singular craving for food in these cases, even when the gastric pain is still considerable. I have seen instances in which patients have required strong beef-tea to be regularly given every three hours.

When the gout flies to the head or lungs, we must avoid bleeding if it can be dispensed with; and we should at all events first try the effect of strong revulsive means.

Acute rheumatism never occurs in advanced life; my remarks will, therefore, be confined to the *chronic* form of the disease, or, as it is often termed, *rheumatic gout*. The joints are the parts affected, there being either effusion into them, or the textures entering into their composition being thickened by some abnormal deposit; and these changes extend so as to affect the extremities of the bones and the cartilages. When the structure of the joints is not permanently altered, we may always hope that treatment will afford considerable relief. The internal treatment consists in the administration of sulphur, guaiacum, Dover's powder, iodide of potassium, &c. Local applications are more effective than internal treatment. When there is much pain, the affected joint may be blistered, and the raw surface sprinkled with a little morphia. In other cases we may try blistering alone, or the application of tincture of iodine.* Warm salt bath, sulphur baths, and corrosive sublimate baths (increasing in strength from two drachms to an ounce for each bath, and continued daily, or every second day, till the gums are slightly affected) have been strongly advocated. The two former may be always tried; the use of the third requires some caution. There is far more power in diligent friction and in

---

* The following formula yields a good tincture for this purpose:—℞. Iodinii ℨi. Potassii iodidi ℨss. Spirit. Rect. ℨi. Misce.

the warm douche than is generally supposed; but great patience is required, and their use is too often abandoned because no immediate effects are perceived.

There is no disease in which mineral waters are more likely to be serviceable, when every thing else has failed, than chronic rheumatism. The Buxton waters are the best in this country; and those who are precluded from visiting the more remote springs of Vichy, Ems, Wiesbaden, and Marienbad,* would do well to try their effects;† but in no instance should a patient use mineral waters, internally or externally, without the advice and concurrence of his physician. Neither is there any disease in which a residence in a warm climate is more beneficial; Rome and Nice are, perhaps, the most eligible situations in Europe. A complete dress of flannel next the skin must always be insisted on; and the diet should not be too low, but such as best to promote the general health.

Muscular rheumatism is an affection that daily presents itself in one form or other to the notice of the physician. It is almost invariably produced by exposure to cold; is often confined to a single muscle, or set of muscles, usually those most directly exposed; and is characterized by local pain, much aggravated by motion, but seldom attended by swelling or heat. The general health is usually unaffected.

The most common forms of muscular rheumatism are lumbago, pleurodynia, and stiff neck, or crick of the neck, as it is sometimes termed. A long chapter might easily be written on the treatment of these forms of muscular rheumatism, but the cases in which they do not yield at once to the thermic treatment are so extremely rare, that it seems unnecessary to enter into the subject. Persons liable to these affections should always avoid cold and wet; they must be especially careful not to lie on damp grass, nor to sit in draughts, or in any way to ex-

---

* These are the most celebrated mineral waters for the cure of gout and chronic rheumatism. At Vichy and Ems there are hot alkaline waters, at Wiesbaden there are hot salt baths, and at Marienbad aperient salines. None can tell so well as the resident physician whether the waters are suitable in individual cases.

† Dr. Robertson of Buxton has published a pamphlet on the use of these waters, which will well repay perusal. In visiting Buxton patients have the advantage of consulting a physician whose admirable work "on Gout" has constituted him a high authority in that and kindred diseases, such as chronic rheumatism.

pose themselves to a chill. They should always wear flannel next the skin, and they cannot medicinally counteract the rheumatic tendency better than by regulating the bowels, and ensuring a due action of the skin by using the electuary prescribed in the note to page 188.

APPENDIX.

ON THE

THERMIC TREATMENT OF LUMBAGO

AND OTHER FORMS OF CHRONIC MUSCULAR RHEUMATISM,

SCIATICA AND OTHER FORMS OF NEURALGIA,

PARALYSIS,

&c. &c.

'Οκόσα φάρμακα οὐκ ἰῆται, σίδηρος ἰῆται ὅσα σίδηρος οὐκ ἰῆται, πῦρ ἰῆται· ὅσα δὲ πῦρ οὐκ ἰῆται, ταῦτα χρὴ νομίζειν ἀνίατα.

ΙΠΠΟΚΡΑΤΟΥΣ ΑΦΟΡΙΣΜΟΙ.

My intention in writing this Appendix is to assist in extending the use of a form of counter-irritation, which I have found of the greatest value in my own practice, and which is comparatively unknown to the great mass of the profession. It consists essentially in the instantaneous application of a flat iron button, gently heated in a spirit-lamp, to the skin. It is an operation completed in a few seconds, productive of little or no pain, immediate in its effects, and altogether incapable of injuring the patient. I believe that the merit of introducing this form of counter-irritation is due to the late Sir Anthony Carlisle, who early in the year 1826 published a letter, addressed to Sir Gilbert Blane, " On Blisters, Rubefacients, and Escharotics, describing the employment of an instrument adapted to effect those several purposes," and in the November number of the Philosophical Magazine addressed a letter to the editor on the same subject. In 1829 M. Mayor, of Lausanne, published a small work " sur la cautérisation avec le marteau," in which he shows that by means of this instrument the effect either of a mustard-poultice, or of a blister, or even of the moxa, may be instantaneously produced. Trousseau subsequently published an account of his experiments with Mayor's hammer, and there, so far as I know, the matter ended, till Dr. Corrigan, about three years ago, published an account of some cases very successfully treated by nearly similar means. My attention had long been directed to the comparative value of the counter-irritants in ordinary use, and I took the earliest opportunity of putting Dr. Corrigan's practice to the test. In the mode of application I differ slightly from him; but the difference is so comparatively unimportant, that I am desirous it should be fully understood that I claim no originality in the matter. As Dr. Corrigan makes no reference to the writings of Carlisle or Mayor, it may be fairly concluded that he was unacquainted with their works. The instrument that I employ is shorter and more portable than that recommended by Corrigan. The button, which is about half an inch in diameter, and a quarter of an inch in thickness, is connected by an iron shank, with a small wooden handle. The whole instrument resembles a very small hammer. The shank is curved nearly at a right angle, at about half an inch from the upper surface of the button. On heating the button, which is effected in about a quarter of a minute by the flame of a spirit-lamp, I place the end of the fore-finger on the curve; when the heat becomes uncomfortable to the finger the instrument is ready for use. Dr. Corrigan's mode of applying it is to touch the surface of the part affected at intervals of half an inch, as lightly and rapidly as possible. I have usually found more service from very lightly drawing the flat surface of the heated button over the affected part, so as to act on a greater extent of surface. The cuticle is never raised, and the only visible effect is a slight degree of local redness, either in lines, according to my plan, or in circular patches if Corrigan's directions are followed. In his paper he relates a case of paralysis of the upper and lower extremities cured by applying the button daily for about three weeks along the spine, thighs, and legs; cases of lumbago and other forms of muscular rheumatism, of sciatica, of neuralgia of the fifth, and paralysis of the seventh pair of nerves.

I now proceed to give a few particulars of some of the cases in which I have found it especially serviceable.

LUMBAGO.

CASE I.—J. A., aged forty, an omnibus conductor, of healthy appearance, and good muscular development. Had frequently suffered from lumbago for several years past. Caught a severe cold in February, but continued his ordinary avocation for some days, till one morning, on attempting to rise, the pain was so severe, that, to use his own expression, he " was obliged to hollow out." He then became a patient at the Western General Dispensary, and remained for upwards of two months under the care of one of my colleagues, who found all the ordinary treatment unavailing in removing the lumbar pains, and knowing that I was engaged in investigating the therapeutic value of the thermic treatment, kindly consented to his being transferred to me. After two applications of the iron at intervals of two days, he said he felt himself fit to resume his work. I met him about a month afterwards, when he told me he had felt no return of the pain since he had previously seen me.

CASE II.—William Gaulton, aged thirty-three, a cab-driver. I first saw him on the 14th of July. He states that he has been liable for some years to rheumatic pains in various parts of the body; at present he complains of no pain except in the loins. Cannot trace this pain to any particular exposure to wet, but thinks he slightly strained himself about a fortnight previously in a fall from the box of his cab. Bowels habitually costive, and subject to piles. Prescribed confection of senna with sulphur, and applied the hammer freely over the loins. On the 16th he informed me that he had experienced *no pain whatever* since his previous visit, but was anxious to have a second application of the hammer as a matter of precaution.

CASE III.—Richard Oliver, aged thirty-four, a baker, subject to lumbago and the chronic cough to which persons in his trade are always liable from the constant irritation produced by the inhalation of particles of flour, consulted me on the 3d of May. The least motion of the body, as for instance, the effort of coughing, gave rise to agonizing pain in the loins; and the peculiar care and caution he observed on sitting down, and on rising from his chair, showed that he was not over-drawing the description of his sufferings. There was frontal headache; his tongue was foul, and his bowels costive; there was a feeling of constriction of the chest, and pain along the whole course of the back, but far the most intense in the lumbar region. I applied the hammer freely over the loins, and upwards along the sides of the spine, and prescribed an emetic, to be followed by a pretty brisk purgative on the following morning.

On the 5th he felt much better; there was less cough, the tongue was comparatively clean, and the bowels had been freely moved. There was, however, still considerable pain in the loins, although much less severe than when I first saw him. The hammer was applied on the 7th and the 10th. On the 12th I dismissed him as cured, and he returned to his work.

CASE IV.*—James M——, aged 40, was first seen on the 5th of May;

* This case occurred in the practice of Dr. M'Cormack, of Rathmullen. I give it

he was then suffering from a severe attack of lumbago, to which he has been a martyr for the last four or five years, so constantly recurring, that he was obliged, about a year ago, to give up his occupation as a fisherman; he has constantly worn a pitch-plaster. The present attack has lasted seven days; he has used several applications, such as warm stupes, liniments of turpentine, &c., but without the least relief. The hammer was applied in about a hundred places along the spine, across the loins, down as far as the sacrum. The rapidity of the relief was extraordinary. To the astonishment of the neighbours who had crowded in to see the operation, he got up and walked about, almost free from pain, while only a few minutes previously he was bent double, and unable to rise off his chair. In a day or two after, fearing he was getting a return of the attack, he requested that the operation might be repeated; this was done, and from that day to this (Nov. 16) he has never had a day's illness from it, although, for the last five years he had scarcely known a week's freedom from pain.

I have notes of numerous other cases in which the relief to patients with confirmed lumbago has been as speedy and as complete as in those I have narrated. Persons who have been for years tortured with this disease, and have been cupped and blistered time after time, with at best only very temporary and partial relief, have been, in several cases, *instantaneously* (I use the word in its literal sense) cured by this application; and I have never met with an instance in which it did not completely yield to three or four of these trivial operations. I call them trivial, for my patients have universally told me that the heat of the hammer caused them far less severe pain than they suffered from the disease. A medical friend, on whom Dr. Corrigan used it, " merely knew that a not disagreeable smarting or heating sensation was suddenly produced." Its extreme superiority over blisters is probably dependent on the suddenness of its action.

OTHER FORMS OF MUSCULAR RHEUMATISM.

CASE V.—Mary G., aged thirty-eight, consulted me on the 8th of

---

because I know that every practitioner is apt, even unconsciously, to attach undue importance to any favourite mode of treatment he may be pursuing, and that the evidence of another person is, *cæteris paribus*, of more real value than his own. See Dr. M'Cormack's cases, illustrating the success of this form of counter-irritation, in *The Lancet*, Dec. 5th, 1846.

November. From her account it would appear that for the last fortnight she had been suffering from rheumatic pain in the right side. This pain, however, gradually disappeared, when two days ago she was seized with a severe pain in the right shoulder, extending to the point of insertion of the deltoid muscle. There was also pain of a less severe character in the inner side of the arm. She had never previously suffered from rheumatism. The arm was supported by a sling, to prevent any action of the muscles, and the pain was so excessive, that she was quite unable, without my assistance, to remove the dress sufficiently to expose the affected part. The hammer was freely applied, and she was desired to call on me the following morning.

On the 9th she informed me that the pain had entirely disappeared immediately after the application, but had slightly reappeared in the morning at the spot where she had previously felt it most severely; it was now confined within the limits of a circle not larger than a crown-piece. She could now move the arm with comparative ease. The hammer was applied over and around the painful spot.

On the 10th there was merely a little tenderness at the spot which was yesterday painful. She no longer wore the sling. She expressed herself as feeling perfectly recovered. I thought it most prudent to make another application, to which she willingly consented, and told her to see me the following morning, if there was any feeling of discomfort in the arm. Not having called since, I conclude that there was no relapse.

I have notes of several cases in which rheumatism of the deltoid muscle yielded to a single application. Dr. M'Cormack also gives the case of a lad, aged seventeen years, who had been much exposed to wet and hardship, and came to him " complaining of a severe pain in the right shoulder joint, extending from it to below the insertion of the deltoid muscle, which, as long as he refrains from severe labour, gives him not much annoyance; but after a hard day's ploughing or digging, or a long walk (he being in the habit of swinging his arms about very much) the pain becomes most intense, and he becomes unable to raise the arm to his head from a deficiency of muscular power." He was cured by a single application.

I have tried this treatment in several cases of crick in the neck, and invariably found the pain removed by a single application. I select the following as a fair illustration of the success of the thermic treatment in this form of rheumatism.

CASE VI.—James Brown, aged about thirty-five, a mechanic, had come a considerable distance from the country in a third-class railway carriage the day before I saw him. He states that he felt a draft upon the back of his neck during a great part of his journey, but went to bed perfectly well, except that he felt generally chilly. On waking he found that his head was considerably drawn downwards, and to the left side, and that any attempt to make it resume its normal position was accompanied with intense pain. He was much alarmed and consulted a chemist in the neighbourhood, who advised him to apply to me. On examination I found that the pain, on slightly moving the head, was confined almost entirely to the position of the sterno-cleido-mastoid muscle. I drew the surface of the hammer about twenty times in a direction parallel to the fibres of that muscle, and concluded by touching the surrounding surface. The whole process occupied less than half a minute, and at its termination he was able to move the head freely in all directions without the least pain.

The following case shows the utility of this treatment in a different class of affections:—

CASE VII.—J. B., aged about twenty-four years, consulted me during the past summer. He states that about six or seven months ago he had a fall, and that the wrist of the right arm was considerably sprained in consequence of the whole weight of his body being thrown on the palm and fingers of the hand. The effect of the fall soon apparently disappeared, but about two or three months afterwards he began to feel a loss of power in the fingers; the sensation remaining unaffected. He mentions, by way of illustration, that in writing, the pen often slips from his hand, and that though he feels it going, he has not the power to retain it. On examination I found a decided loss of power in the flexor muscles. I applied the thermic treatment, at intervals of two or three days, along the course of these muscles from the wrist upwards, for about three weeks, by which time they had regained their former tone. I was led to try it in this instance from the similarity it presented to certain cases successfully treated by Drs. Corrigan and M'Cormack. I have no doubt that many cases of this sort, which I formerly treated with the galvano-magnetic current, would have recovered more rapidly under the thermic treatment.

SCIATICA AND OTHER NEURALGIC PAINS.

In my remarks on the treatment of Sciatica (see page 124) I mentioned that if I were compelled to adhere to a single remedy, it would unquestionably be to that which I am now advocating, and I likewise pointed out the advantage it possessed over all other forms of treatment. The following cases show the efficacy in this painful and distressing affection.

CASE VIII.—William Smith, aged about thirty-five, was sent to me last March by his employer. Is a common labourer, and has been engaged lately in draining, an occupation that exposes him to much wet and cold. About five weeks ago, he states that, after having worked the greater part of the day in wet clothes, he caught a severe cold, and felt considerable pain in the loins. The pain extended to the left buttock, and from thence gradually down to the foot. He thinks it was about a fortnight "working its way down," along the whole course of the thigh and foot. He has continued to suffer all the ordinary symptoms of lumbago associated with very severe sciatica, without, however, any serious disturbance of the general health. The pain is stated to be most severe at night; often preventing him from obtaining any rest. It is also much aggravated by the least motion of the foot or leg. On examining the limb I found that pressure with the finger excited great pain in the regions of the sacro-iliac articulation, of the trochanter major, in the popliteal space, and behind and rather below the malleolus. In fact every twig of the sciatic nerve seemed more or less involved. Having first sketched in ink the lines, along which I meant to apply the hammer, I made him lie down, and drew it rapidly over the direction indicated, from above downwards, besides freely applying it to the loins. He expressed himself considerably relieved, and evidently did not dread moving the leg as he had previously done. I prescribed a little confection of senna and sulphur, and gave particular directions that he should guard against any chill.

On seeing him three days afterwards, I found that the pain had slightly returned every night, but that it was not so severe, and that during the day the sensation was hardly deserving the name of pain. There was little pain excited on pressure, except in the vicinity of the trochanter major.

Three more operations, at intervals of two or three days, each slighter and more limited than the last, completely removed the affection. Although not a case of long standing, it was one of the most severe I ever witnessed.

While lumbago and other forms of muscular rheumatism are often completely removed by a single application, I have usually found that entirely to eradicate sciatica, requires three, and occasionally more. The following case in Dr. M'Cormack's practice shows, however, that one application occasionally suffices, even in severe forms of the disease.

CASE IX.—George M——, aged forty-five, a pensioner of very intemperate habits, came under Dr. M'Cormack's care on the 10th of December. "He has been for some days complaining of flying rheumatism, which he greatly aggravated by his intemperance, and by being constantly exposed, while drunk, to the severity of the weather. On the Sunday following his first application to me for relief, I was requested to go in a great hurry to see him, by his wife, who declared he was on the point of death, roaring with pain. On my arriving at his house, I found him in bed, not able to turn or move in the smallest degree from the agony he was suffering in the right hip, and down the leg to the toes; he was unable to close an eye the previous night, pulse quick, full and incompressible; skin hot and dry; had not yet recovered from his previous debauch. I at once proceeded to apply the firing-iron over the hip, lumbar region, and down the course of the sciatic nerve, as far as the knee. I made about one hundred applications altogether; the effect produced was positively miraculous. I had scarcely laid down the iron when he declared he was quite well: he turned round in the bed with the greatest ease, and bent the thigh on the hip, which before he was unable to do; he was able to sit up at the fire that evening, and the next day (to the astonishment of those who saw him on the previous one, as they thought dying), he was able to go out with merely the aid of a stick. In three or four days after this, having had another drinking bout, and become exposed to wet, he came to me to have the firing reapplied. Since that period till the time of his death, which took place early in June, from phthisis, he never had the slightest return of the complaint, although constantly drunk, and exposed to much cold and wet."

I shall give one more case of sciatica, and this is one that I consider particularly valuable, because the patient is a member of the profession. In the following letter to Dr. Corrigan, he describes his own case, and the benefit he derived from the thermic treatment.

CASE X.—"Early in the month of May, 1845, I was rather suddenly attacked with severe pains in the right thigh, extending from the hip to the knee. Having never suffered from any similar affection, and generally having good health, I hoped this pain would have yielded to rest, and the warm bath, which last remedy I had recourse to after a week's suffering. This was not the case, I only obtained temporary relief; the pain now became more fixed, and was so increased in intensity, that I could not walk the shortest distance without being obliged to stand at every twenty or thirty paces to obtain ease, which I did the moment I stopped. The entire of the thigh participated in the affection, but I felt the pain principally along the course of the sciatic and anterior crural nerves; I could not endure to lie on the affected side, as doing so considerably increased the pain. I continued to suffer in this manner for a period of six months, during which time I had recourse to the usual remedies of warm baths, frictions, strong stimulating liniments, hyd. potassæ and morphia in combination, tinct. aconit., electro-magnetism, and all without any effect more than temporary relief. Changes of temperature produced very little, if any effect. I then applied to Dr. Corrigan, who immediately applied the hot iron, from which application I received considerable relief, so much so, that in two days I was more free from pain than I had been from the entire period since the commencement of the attack. The first day that the last remedy was tried, I had a distance of about half a mile to walk to Dr. Corrigan's house, which occupied me nearly an hour, being obliged to stand at least fifty times to obtain relief. I did not go to Dr. Corrigan until after a week, and on my second visit I was able to walk the same distance without once resting. After about eight applications of the hot iron in the space of four or five weeks, I became perfectly free from pain, now being able to walk a considerable distance without much inconvenience, I discontinued my attendance on Dr. Corrigan. Several weeks passed without my being at all troubled by any return of the pain; but within the last fortnight I have had some temporary attacks. I think it right to say I feel satisfied that if I had continued the application of this remedy some time longer, the cure would have been complete."

I trust that the cases I have given will be regarded as furnishing sufficient evidence of the singular efficacy of the thermic treatment in a class of diseases which are usually regarded as of a most intractable and obstinate character. I may add that I have successfully applied it in spinal irritation, in various painful manifestations of hysteria, and in many forms of neuralgia; and I cannot conclude without again expressing my conviction that the practitioner who will give the thermic treatment a fair trial, will not readily abandon a remedial agent by which human suffering can be so easily and rapidly alleviated.

INDEX.

	Page
Ablution, Importance of	46
Abscess near the rectum	147
Acne rosacea	190
Aconite, its use in affections of the heart	159
ALDERSON, his cases of cancer (note)	134
Ale, its use as a beverage	42
Anæmia of the brain	104
Animal heat, necessity of supporting it	44
Anointing, Probable value of	47
Anus, Hemorrhage from the	139
,, Itching of the	143
,, Mucous discharge from the	141
,, Paralysis of its sphincter	147
,, Tumour of the	140
Aphthous eruptions of the mouth	127
Apoplexy and hepatic disease, Connexion between	155
,, Danger after an attack of	107
,, Meningeal	108
,, Premonitory symptoms of	105
Appetite, Loss of	126
Arteries, Alterations in the	35
Asses milk, How to prepare artificial	41
Asthma	86
Atmospheric influences	44
Atrophy, Senile (note)	54
Bathing, Importance of	46
Bed, Patent spring	ix.
Beef-tea, Liebig's directions for making	65
Beer, its use as a beverage	42
Bibliography	x.
Birds, the most wholesome	41
Bladder, Catarrh of the	169
,, Chronic inflammation of the	168
,, Hemorrhage from the	171
,, Irritability of the	170, 176
,, Paralysis of the	162
,, Spasm of its neck	167
Blisters, their value	57

	Page
Blood, sources of its impurity	35
Blood-letting, cautions regarding	56
Blood-spitting	95
Boiling-meat, Liebig's rules for	39
Bougie, Rectum	146
Bowels, Attention to the	50
,, Regulation of the	42
,, Relaxation of the	52
Brain, Alterations in the	31
,, Anæmia of the	104
,, Deficiency of energy in the	104
,, Hyperæmia of the	103
,, Softening of the	110
Brandy, Occasional use of	43
Breakfast, Rules regarding	43
BRIGHT's Disease	171
Bronchitis, Senile	78
Bronchorrhœa, Chronic	82
Camphor, its value	x. 59
Cancer of the stomach	134
Capillaries, Alteration in the	35
Carbuncled face	190
Catarrh, Common	82
,, of the bladder	169
Changes occurring in the system in advanced life	27
Chloroform	ix. 58
Cholera, English	132
Cigarettes for Asthma	91
Climacteric disease	60
Climate, Therapeutic value of	46
Clothing, Importance of warm	44
Collodion, a remedy for cutaneous diseases	194
Concretion in the kidney, symptoms of	182
Constipation	127
Consumption, Pulmonary	93
Cookery, Chemistry of	39
Cough, Dyspeptic	131
Death, Causes of, in aged persons	27
,, No fear of, in aged persons	27
Deposits, Urinary	172
Diarrhœa, A natural form of	52

INDEX.

	Page
Digestive Organs, Changes in the	34
Dilatation of the heart	162
Diminished nutrition, Causes of	35
Dinner, Rules regarding	43
Discharges, Danger of checking	59
Diseases, Relative fatality of	66
Doses required in advanced life	57
Drink, Articles of	42
Dropsy of the abdomen	152
,, Organic	154
,, from disease of the heart	161
,, from disease of the kidneys	173
Dyspepsia, Acute, atonic	129
,, Causes of, in old persons	35
,, Follicular gastric	130
,, Senile	129
Dysphagia	128
Eating, Rules regarding	44
Ecthyma	190
Eczema	186
Eggs, as an article of Diet	41
English Cholera	132
Epidermis, Alterations in the	33
Epochs of declining life	26
Erysipelas	187
Erythema	187
Excretions, Importance of attention to the	50
Exercise, Importance of	48
Expectoration common in old persons	34
Fainting	158
Fatality of different diseases	66
Fish, The most wholesome	41
Flatulence	126
Friction, Importance of	47
Fruits, Caution regarding	42
Gall-stones	148
Gangrene, Senile	195
Gastritis of aged persons	133
,, Gouty	133
,, Ulcerative	134
GLAISHER, his directions for using the dry and wet bulb thermometer in the sick-room	82
Gout, Acute	198
,, Chronic	205
,, Erratic	207
,, Retrocedent	207
Gravel	178
Hæmaturia	170
Hæmoptysis	96
Hemorrhage, Uterine	186

	Page
Hemorrhoidal discharge	139
,, tumours	140
HALFORD on Climacteric Disease	61
Head-symptoms	103
Heart, Alterations in the	35
,, Anatomy of the aged	160
,, Functional Diseases of the	156
,, Neuralgia of the	159
,, Organic Diseases of the	159
Herpes	187
HOURMANN and DECHAMBRE, their researches	28
Hydrocele, treatment of	59
Hydrothorax	92
Hygrometrical precautions	82
Hyperæmia of the brain	103
Icterus senilis	150
Impetigo	190
Incontinence of urine	170
Inflammation	55
,, of the bladder, a cause of retention of urine	167
Influenza	96
Insanity, Various forms of	117
Insulation of different organs	34
Interference, Propriety or danger of	55
Itching of the anus	143
Jaundice, Senile	150
Kidney-disease, secondary on enlarged prostate	170
Lichen	193
LIEBIG, his Chemistry of Cookery	39
Liver, Diseases of the	148
Long Life, How to attain a	37
Luncheon, Rules regarding	43
Lungs of aged persons, Peculiarities in the	28
,, Deposits in the	30
,, Inflammation of the	68
Marasmus, Senile	64
Meal-times, The best	38
Meats, Best kinds of	40
,, To boil	39
Medicines, the form of their administration	56
Meningeal Apoplexy	108
Meningitis	115
Mental diseases of advanced life	117
,, faculties, their decline	119
Mercury, Remarks on	58
Metals, inapplicable in advanced life	58
Milk, as an article of diet	41
Moisture of the sick-room, Importance of attending to	81

INDEX.

	Page
Mortality, influence of seasons on	45
Mucous Flux of the aged	82
Mutton chops, How to cook	40
Narcotics, Cautions regarding	58
Nerves, Painful affections of the	127
Neuralgia	121
„ of the heart	159
Non-interference	59
Nutrition, causes of diminished	35
Œdema of the lungs	93
Œsophagus, Stricture of the	128
Organs of circulation, Alterations in	35
Organic Diseases of the heart	159
Oysters, a good food for invalids	42
Ozone, the probable cause of influenza	100
Palpitation	156
Paralysed limbs, Local treatment of	107
Paralysis of the bladder	163
„ sphincter ani	147
Passive congestion, its effects on the brain	104
Pemphigus	189
Pennock, his investigations	30
Perspiration, Excessive	50
Phthisis, Case of prolonged	94
Piles	140
Pills, Objection to the use of	57
Pneumonia	68
Prostate gland, Enlargement of	164
„ „ Varicosity of	167
Prurigo	191
„ podicis	143
„ senilis	175
Puddings, Rules regarding	42
Pulmonary consumption	93
Pulse, Deceptive character of the	55
„ Remarks on the	36
Purgatives, Occasional injury from	51
Psoriasis	193
Pyrosis	129
Reaction, its absence in old age	54
Rectum, Abscess near the	147
„ bougie, remarks on the	146
„ Congestion of the	137
„ Diseases of the	137
„ Inflammation of the	142
„ Stricture of the	144
Reichenbach, the observations of	49
Regular habits, their importance	38
Renovation of power occasionally observed	60
Respiration, Cerebral (note)	106
Respirations, Number of the	30

	Page
Respiratory organs, Changes in the	28
„ system, Diseases of the	68
Retention of urine	162
Rheiocline, The	ix.
Rosy drop	190
Rupia	190
Salts, Caution regarding their use	57
Sciatica	123
Senile Bronchitis	78
„ Dementia	118
„ Dyspepsia	129
„ Gangrene	195
„ Jaundice	150
„ Marasmus	64
Senses, Alteration in the	32
Sex, its influence on the constitution	54
Sexual feeling, Augmentation of	186
„ „ Diminution of	186
Skin, danger of checking its action	50
„ Diseases of the	187
„ Importance of attention to the	46
Skull, its alterations in advanced life	31
Sleep, How to obtain	ix.
„ Rules regarding	48
Sleeplessness, a frequent subject of complaint	48
„ How to obviate	ix. 49
Softening, Cerebral	110
Soup, Liebig's directions for making	39
Spasm of the neck of the bladder	167
Stimulants, their importance	59
Stone in the bladder	182
„ Possibility of dissolving	184
Stomach, Cancer of the	134
Stricture of the œsophagus	128
„ „ rectum	144
„ „ urethra	165, 168
Straining at the water closet, Danger of	51
Stramonium, its uses in asthma	90
Sulphur, a valuable remedy	58
Surgical operations, Increased danger of	59
Swallowing, Pain or difficulty in	128
Syme, his treatment of senile gangrene	197
Sympathy between different organs, its absence	34
Syncope	158
Tea, Rules regarding	43
Temperature, its importance in surgical operations	124
Thermic treatment, its importance	124
Thermometer, dry and wet bulb, its importance	81

16

INDEX.

	Page		Page
Tic Douloureux	122	Urine, Incontinence of	170
Tonics	59	,, Retention of	162
Turtle, a good food for invalids	41	Uterine hemorrhage	186
Transpiration, Cutaneous	50		
		Vegetables, The most wholesome	42
Ulcers of the legs	194	Venesection, Cautions regarding	56
Urinary deposits	53, 177		
,, functions, importance of attention to the	52	Wakefulness, To prevent	ix. 49
		Wasting	64
,, organs, Diseases of	162	Water-brash	129
Urine, Acrid	175	Water on the chest	92
,, Albuminous	171	Wines	43
,, Bloody	170		
,, danger of retaining it too long	52	Zymotic, Meaning of the term (note)	96

AGING AND OLD AGE

An Arno Press Collection

(Armstrong, John). **The Art of Preserving Health.** 1744

Canstatt, Carl. **Die Krankheiten des Hoheren Alters Und Ihre Heilung.** 1839

Carlisle, Anthony. **An Essay on the Disorders of Old Age, and on the Means for Prolonging Human Life.** 1818

Cavan, Ruth Shonle, et al. **Personal Adjustment in Old Age.** 1949

Charcot, J(ean) M(artin). **Clinical Lectures on Senile and Chronic Diseases.** 1881

Cheyne, George. **An Essay of Health and Long Life.** 1724

Child, Charles. **Sensecence and Rejuvenescence.** 1915

Cicero, M(arcus) T(ullius). **Cato Major.** 1744

(Cohausen, Johann Heinrich). **Hermippus Redivivus.** 1771

Cornaro, Luigi. **The Art of Living Long.** 1917

Cowdry, E. V., ed. **Problems of Ageing.** 1939

Cumming, Elaine and William E. Henry. **Growing Old.** 1961

Day, George E. **A Practical Treatise on the Domestic Management and Most Important Diseases of Advanced Life.** 1849

Department for the Aging, City of New York. **Older Women in the City.** 1979

Floyer, John. **Medicina Gerocomica.** 1724

Gruman, Gerald J., ed. **The "Fixed Period" Controversy.** 1979

Gruman, Gerald J., ed. **Roots of Modern Gerontology and Geriatrics.** 1979

(Hufeland, Christoph Wilhelm). **Art of Prolonging Life.** 1854

Jameson, Thomas. **Essays on the Changes of the Human Body at Its Different Ages.** 1811

Kirk, Hyland Clare. **When Age Grows Young.** 1888

Kleemeier, Robert W., ed. **Aging and Leisure.** 1961

Lessius, Leonard and Lewis Cornaro. **A Treatise of Health and Long Life With the Future Means of Attaining It.** 1743

MacKenzie, James. **The History of Health, and the Art of Preserving It.** 1760

Martin, Lillien J(ane) and Clare de Gruchy. **Sweeping the Cobwebs.** 1933

Minot, Charles S. **The Problem of Age, Growth, and Death.** 1908

Nascher, I(gnatz) L(eo). **Geriatrics.** 1914

Pearl, Raymond and Ruth DeWitt Pearl. **The Ancestry of the Long-Lived.** 1934

Ramon y Cajal, S(antiago). **El Mundo Visto a Los Ochenta Anos.** 1934

de Ropp, Robert S. **Man Against Aging.** 1960

Stieglitz, Edward J. **The Second Forty Years.** 1946

Sweetser, William. **Human Life.** 1867

Thoms, William J. **Human Longevity.** 1873

Tibbitts, Clark, ed. **Living Through the Older Years.** 1949

Tolstoy, Leo. **Last Diaries.** 1960

Vercors (pseud. Jean Bruller). **The Insurgents.** 1956

Warthin, Aldred Scott. **Old Age.** 1929